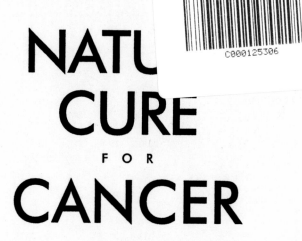

NATURAL CURE

FOR

CANCER

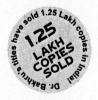

DR. H. K. BAKHRU

NATIONALLY ACCLAIMED NATUROPATH

JAICO PUBLISHING HOUSE

Ahmedabad Bangalore Bhopal Bhubaneswar Chennai
Delhi Hyderabad Kolkata Lucknow Mumbai

Published by Jaico Publishing House
A-2 Jash Chambers, 7-A Sir Phirozshah Mehta Road
Fort, Mumbai - 400 001
jaicopub@jaicobooks.com
www.jaicobooks.com

NATURE CURE FOR CANCER
ISBN 978-81-7992-763-2

First Jaico Impression: 2008
Sixth Jaico Impression: 2012

Printed by
Repro India Limited
Plot No. 50/2, T.T.C. MIDC Industrial Area
Mahape, Navi Mumbai - 400 710

OTHER BOOKS BY DR. H.K. BAKHRU

1. A Complete Handbook Of Nature Cure
2. Diet Cure For Common Ailments
3. A Handbook Of Natural Beauty
4. Nature Cure For Children
5. Naturopathy For Longevity
6. Healing Through Natural Foods
7. Indian Spices And Condiments As Natural Healers
8. Foods That Heal
9. Herbs That Heal
10. Natural Home Remedies For Common Ailments
11. Vitamins That Heal
12. Conquering Diabetes Naturally

ABOUT THE AUTHOR

Dr. H.K. Bakhru enjoys a countrywide reputation as an expert naturopath and a prolific writer. His well-researched articles on nature cure, health, nutrition and herbs appears regularly in various newspapers and magazines and bear the stamp of authority.

A diploma holder in Naturopathy, all his current 13 books on nature cure, nutrition and herbs titled, 'A Complete Handbook Of Nature Cure', 'Diet Cure For Common Ailments', 'A Handbook Of Natural Beauty', 'Nature Cure For Children', 'Naturopathy For Longevity', 'Healing Through Natural Foods', 'Indian Spices And Condiments As Natural Healers', 'Foods That Heal', 'Herbs That Heal', 'Natural Home Remedies For Common Ailments', 'Vitamins That Heal' and 'Conquering Diabetes Naturally' have been highly appreciated by the public and repeatedly reprinted. His first-named book has been awarded first prize in the category 'Primer on Naturopathy for Healthy Living' by the jury of judges at the 'Book Prize Award', an autonomous body under govt. of India, Ministry of Health.

Dr. Bakhru began his career with the Indian Railways, with a first class first postgraduate degree in History from Lucknow University, in 1949. He retired in October 1984, as the Chief Public Relations Officer of the Central Railway in Mumbai, having to his credit 35 years of distinguished service in the Public Relations Organizations of the Indian Railways and the Railway Board.

An associate member of the All India Alternative Medical Practitioner's Association and a member of the Nature Cure Practitioners' Guild, in Mumbai, Dr. Bakhru has made extensive studies of natural methods of treating diseases and herbalism. He has been honoured with the 'Lifetime Achievement Award', 'Gem of Alternative Medicines' award and a gold medal in Diet Therapy by the Indian Board of Alternative Medicines, Calcutta, in recognition of his dedication and outstanding contributions in the field of Alternative Medicines. The Board, which is affiliated to the Open International University for Complementary Medicines, established under World Health Organisation and recognized by the United Nations Peace University, has also appointed him as its Honorary Advisor. Dr. Bakhru has also been honoured by Nature Cure Practitioners' Guild, Bombay with the Nature Cure Appreciation Award for his services in Naturopathy.

Dr. Bakhru has founded a registered Public Charitable Trust, known a D.H. Bakhru Foundation, to help the poor and needy. He has been donating Rs. 25,000 every year to this trust from his income as writer and author.

CONTENTS

Sore Mouth : Gargling with lemon juice and
water, mouth wash with salt and baking soda

PREFACE

In my naturopathic practice of over 15 years, I have come across several cases of cancer. Some of the patients who came for consultation were in the initial stages of the disease, while others were at an advanced stage. Those in early stages were greatly helped by my prescription of dietary treatment, suggested changes in lifestyle, by the use of specific foods, found helpful in controlling cancers and other natural methods aimed at strengthening the immune system for healing. However, not much help could be rendered to those in advanced stages, except to make them feel better and comfortable by suggested changes in diet, lifestyle and other natural methods.

In almost all cases of cancer, I have observed that the digestion of the patients 15 completely deranged. They are unable to pass motion without the use of purgatives and enemas. In some cases, where the bowels could be moved, the food would pass through motion as it was eaten, without any digestion. This condition has been brought about by accumulation of excessive morbid matter in the system resulting from wrong feeding habits and faulty style of living for a long period, ultimately leading to cancer. The foremost consideration in any natural treatment for cancer in the beginning is thus, the thorough cleansing of the system through fasting on raw fresh fruit and vegetable juices or an all-fruit diet, with frequent warm water enemas to detoxify the body. After this initial cleansing process, the patient can be greatly helped by adopting sensible diet, based mainly on alkaline raw fruits, and a complete change in the life style.

This book aims at providing detailed information about cancer, its symptoms and their natural remedies, causes, types, their diagnosis and their treatments, both medical as well as natural. It describes how diet can fight cancer and how specific foods, can intervene and halt or retard, the progress of cancer at various stages of its development. For the benefit of those suffering from this disease a treatment chart through natural methods has been included, as a supportive treatment to whatever specialised, medical treatment they are undergoing under expert advice.

DR. H.K. BAKHRU

CANCER: AN INTRODUCTION

The word "Cancer" comes from the Latin word 'Carcinoma' meaning crab. It is the most dreaded disease and refers to all malignant tumours caused by the abnormal growth of a body cell or a group of cells. It is today, the second largest killer in the world, next only to heart ailments. The term covers more than 200 diseases.

Cancer is a chronic degenerative disease, where almost all essential organs are involved in the more advanced cases. The entire metabolism the intestines liver and pancreas, the circulatory apparatus, the kidneys and bile system, the reticuloendothelial and lymphatic system, the central nervous system for most metabolic and motoric purposes, are all severely affected by this disease.

Cancer has been prevalent since ancient times. Hippocrates (460-370 B.C.), the father of medicine, termed it *karkinois,* as the swollen blood vessels going and coming from the tumour mass, give the appearance of the claws of a crab. Sushruta, the ancient medical authority of India, described it as a tumour which would ulcerate and would not cure and "sow its seeds in other parts of the body". Cancer has, however, assumed alarming proportions in modern time and is therefore, called a disease of modern civilization. It is caused by health-destroying eating and living habits. This results in a biochemical imbalance and physical and chemical irritation of the tissues. Carcinogens are present in abundance in today's food, water, air and environment. Carcinogenic substances are also produced within the body as a result of deranged metabolism.

There are billions of cells in the body which, under normal circumstances, develop in a well-organized pattern for the growth of the body and the repair of damaged tissues. Cell, it may be mentioned here, is a basic until of all living things or organisms, which can reproduce itself exactly. When cancer sets in, a group of cells start multiplying suddenly in a haphazard manner and form a lump or tumour. Cancer can spread very rapidly and eventually prove fatal, if not treated properly and in time.

Characteristics of Cancer

Cancer can develop in any organ of the body. The most important characteristic of many cancers is the development of a new growth, a nodule or a tumour in the tissues of their origin. The other features of cancer are that the original tumour or growth has a remarkable tendency to form colonies at some distant parts of the body. This tendency of forming tumours elsewhere in the body makes the disease extremely difficult for satisfactory treatment.

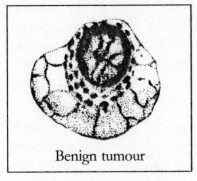
Benign tumour

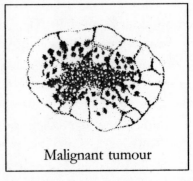
Malignant tumour

There are two types of tumours known as *Benign* and *Malignant*. Only malignant tumours are termed as cancers. They do not have capsules or limiting membrane. They therefore, invade and destroy the tissues in which they occur.

They reproduce their cells in a disorderly and uncontrolled way. The cells are of a more primitive type than the originating tissue. The rate of growth is unusually rapid. They are capable of producing secondary growths in parts of the body remote from the original tumour.

Benign tumours are opposite to malignant growth. They have capsules of fibrous tissues and do not invade normal tissue. They reproduce themselves in orderly ways. The cells resemble the tissue in which they originate. The rate of growth of benign tumour is slow and they stop spontaneously. They do not spread, except by direct extension. They are not fatal, except perhaps in the skull. They only produce ill-effects by occupying space and pressing on adjacent normal tissue.

Spread of Cancer

Cancer, when it has become established in any tissue, spreads in various ways. The process by which it spreads is known as Metastasis, in medical parlance. The cancer cells multiply at the site of their origin and form a tumour mass, which may grow gradually and ultimately attain an enormous size. The cells may also penetrate into the surrounding tissues, and gradually destroy them. Some of the cancer cells which are loosely attached to one another, may get detached and be carried by the lymph stream to the regional lymph nodes and later, to the distant organs. There, they grow independently, multiply and reproduce the original growth.

In rare cases, they spread by invading the bloodstream and setting up secondary growth in bones, lungs and particularly, the liver. For instance, cancers of the intestines especially spread to the liver through the portal system of vessels. Cancers arising in the brain do not metastasize, but cancers arising elsewhere metastasize to the brain.

Kinds of Cancer

There are three main kinds of cancer. These are *carcinoma*, *sarcoma* and *leukaemia*. A malignant tumour arising in an epithelial tissue is known as a carcinoma and one arising in connective tissue as a sarcoma. Leukaemia is a malignant condition of the blood in which the bone, marrow and other blood-forming organs over-produce immature or abnormal white cells.

The Greek word for a tumour is *onkos* and the study of neoplasia is known as oncology. Substances known to produce tumours are said to be carcinogenic or oncogenic.

How Cancer differs from Other Diseases

Cancer differs from other diseases in many ways. Several acute and some chronic infections are characterised by symptoms, which are easily recongnised by the patient and his doctor. Similarly, the patient and his relatives can easily recognize the symptoms of metabolic disorders and conditions caused by nutritional deficiencies. But in case of cancer, certain unfavorable circumstances make it difficult for its early detection and treatment. There are not early warning signals like fever and pain to indicate that something is wrong in the body and seek relief. Moreover, the cancer cells are altered normal cells and not foreign to the body.

Incidence of Cancer

Sex does not affect the incidence of the disease. However, proportion of cancer in males and females is roughly 10:12. It also affects the site of growth. In men, cancer is usually found in the intestines, the prostate and the lungs. In women, it occurs mostly in the breast tissues, uterus, gall-bladder and thyroid.

Cancer occurs at all ages, from infancy to old age. There is a close relationship between cancer and aging. In the United States, over one-half of all cancers occur in 11 per cent of the population over the age of 65. At the age of 25, the probability of developing cancer within five years is one in 700, while at the age of 65, it is one in 14. The peak incidence and mortality of cancer is in the 60-70 age range.

Although deaths attributable to cancer decrease from 30 per cent at age 50 to 10 per cent or less at age 85, this is largely due to rapid increase in death due to other causes with advancing age, and not due to non-prevalence of cancer. Despite the marked increase in cardiovascular related deaths with age, cancer remains the second leading cause of death in those over 65.

In India, the incidence of cancer is the same as that of many people in different parts of the world. Approximately, five lakh new cases of cancer occur every year in this country. According to the Indian Cancer Society, about 1.5 million people suffer from this disease, at any one time. Like other countries, the human life span is increasing in India, so is the incidence of cancer. It is thus, an emerging problem in this country.

However, cancer of some parts of the body are much more frequent among Indians. Cancers of the sex and accessory sex organs account for more than 60 per cent of all cancers in women and hardly five per cent in men. So also, cancers of the mouth, throat and gullet constitute more than half of all cancers in Indian people. Oral cancer and cervix Cancer account for the highest number of cancers in this country.

Cancer is not contagious or infectious. This is clearly evident from the fact that a large number of members of the medical profession and technicians come in close contact and handle cancer tissues in the course of treating patients, but they do not get cancer any more than other sections of the people. No infective agent has so far been detected from cancer tissues.

Detection of Cancer

It is of utmost importance that the cancer is detected in its early stage of development, as it is only in this stage that cancer can be treated with success. Advanced cases of cancer are extremely difficult to treat and usually prove fatal. It is therefore, essential that a healthy person should periodically undergo a careful clinical examination for possible detection of cancer and its early treatment. Persons in the age group in which cancers are most likely to occur should always remember the common sites of cancer and, in case of any suspicion, should consult the specialist about their symptoms.

Diagnosis

The best way of diagnosing cancer is through a process called 'biopsy'. In this process, a piece of suspect tissue is examined and tested under a microscope.

Chance of Recovery

Questions are always asked by laymen regarding recovery from cancer. The answer is, with advances in medical science, and the rapid progress made in natural methods of treating diseases, cancer can be treated successfully if it is detected early and has not spread to other adjoining tissues or to other organs of the body. Cancer in the initial stages can also be controlled effectively through diet and proper selection of foods as well as other natural methods of treatment, described in Chapter-9. The disease usually develops gradually over a long period of time. Latest research studies show that certain specific foods can intervene and checks its progress at various stages of growth.

It may also be mentioned that some cancers are more easily curable than others. For instance, most cancers of lining membranes like the skin, are relatively less malignant and more readily curable than those of the connective tissue and the muscle beneath it.

SYMPTOMS OF CANCER AND THEIR NATURAL REMEDIES

2

There are several types of cancer. The clinical experimental tests conducted during the past several decades have shown that although cancers of different tissues possess several common characteristics, they differ in many respects from one another. These differences vary according to sites of growth, tissues of origin and character of cells which go to make up cancer.

It may be clarified that all tumours are not cancerous. There is a process of cell multiplication and partial or complete differentiation, when cancer starts. However, the newly-developed cancer cells are unresponsive to the cell-restraining mechanism. The tumour cells keep on multiplying until they form a fleshy mass or a new growth, which invades the surrounding normal tissue. This proliferation constitutes the distinctive feature of a cancerous growth and only such tumours with this characteristic, can be termed as a cancer.

The symptoms of cancer vary according to the site of the growth. The main symptoms are tumour or swelling. This is always a sign of danger and one should look on with suspicion, any swelling of the tissues, anywhere in the body. Even a goitre, which is an enlargement of the thyroid gland in the front of the neck, may become malignant at some point.

Besides tumour or swelling, the most common symptoms are as follows:

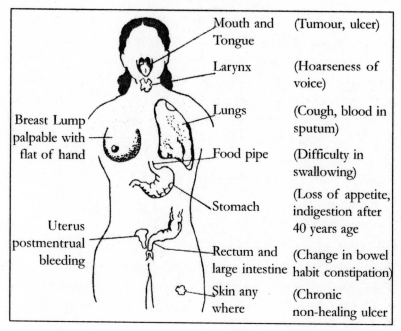

Mouth and Tongue — (Tumour, ulcer)

Larynx — (Hoarseness of voice)

Lungs — (Cough, blood in sputum)

Food pipe — (Difficulty in swallowing)

Stomach — (Loss of appetite, indigestion after 40 years age

Breast Lump palpable with flat of hand

Uterus postmentrual bleeding

Rectum and large intestine — (Change in bowel habit constipation)

Skin any where — (Chronic non-healing ulcer

1. Pain

Pain is usually considered to be one the chief symptoms of cancer, but is not actually a common symptom in most cases of the disease. As many as half the cancers in even an advanced stage, do not cause pain. But where it is present, it may be continuous, gradually increasing in intensity and may become unbearable. Thus, for instance, painless swellings in the breast or in the muscle may indicate an underlying carcinoma or sarcoma, respectively. Lymphomas are usually painless enlargements of lymph nodes or spleen. Space-occupying lesions in the brain will cause symptoms of raised intracranial pressure such as headache, vomiting or visual disturbance.

Natural Remedies: The use of garlic and garlic milk has been found highly beneficial in relieving pain. This vegetable should be cut into small pieces and taken with a teaspoon of honey with each meal. Taken over a period of time, it will yield good results in relieving pain and suffering. Garlic milk can be prepared both in cooked and uncooked states. In the raw state, the uncooked form is more powerful. This milk is prepared by adding the pulp of crushed garlic in uncooked buffalo milk. The proportion is four cloves to 110ml. of milk. Another method is to boil the garlic in milk.

Hot fomentation can also be applied on the painful part of the body to get relief. *The procedure for this application has been explained in chapter 9 on Natural Methods.*

2. Loss of Appetite and Weight

Lack of appetite and consequent loss of weight are other common symptoms of cancer, especially in older people. These may be due to poor appetite, resulting in less intake of food. Moreover, cancer tissues burn excessive energy of the body. Vomiting and diarrhoea, wherever present, also accounts for less absorption of food. Sometimes, the loss of weight occurs so slowly that it is hardly noticed.

Natural Remedies: The use of orange and lime are extremely valuable in controlling loss of appetite. They stimulate the flow of digestive juices, thereby improving digestion and increasing appetite. The use of garlic is also beneficial as it stimulates the digestive tone and improves appetite.

3. Nausea and Vomiting

Nausea and Vomiting are common symptoms after chemotherapy or radiation. Sometimes, they are so severe that they become unbearable.

Natural Remedies: Ginger juice can help in the treatment of this condition. A quarter teaspoon or 15 drops of fresh ginger juice, mixed with half a teaspoon each of fresh lime and mint juices and a teaspoon of honey, constitutes an effective medicine for this purpose. The juice of red beet is another effective remedy for vomiting. About half a cup of the juice, with equal quantity of water, may be taken twice daily. Adding half a teaspoon of lime juice to this juice will increase its medicinal value.

4. Shortness of Breath and Cough

Shortness of breath accompanied by cough, is a very common symptom of cancer, especially lung cancer. Bronchogenic tumours may also cause shortness of breath or cough resulting from partial or complete blockage of an airway.

Natural Remedies: The use of honey is considered valuable in treating shortness of breath. It is said that if a jug of honey is held under the nose of a person suffering from shortness of breath and he inhales the air that comes into contact with the honey, he starts breathing easily and deeply. The effect lasts for about an hour or so. This is because honey contains a mixture of 'higher' alcohol and ethereal oils and the vapours given off by them are beneficial and soothing. Honey, eaten or taken either in milk or water, will also be beneficial in shortness of breath. Relief from cough can be obtained by use of grapes. They tone up the lungs. A cup of grape juice mixed with a teaspoon of honey can be taken with beneficial results in treating this condition.

5. Diarrhoea

Diarrhoea is quite common after treatment of cancer through chemotherapy. Occasionally, it is also a symptom of cancer itself.

Natural Remedies: Buttermilk can be used to control this condition. It helps overcome harmful intestinal flora. It should be taken with a pinch of salt, two or three times daily for treating this condition.

Fenugreek seeds have been used in India for a long time as a natural medicine for diarrhoea and gastrointestinal spasms. Half a teaspoon of these seeds, taken three times a day, often produces quick and marked relief.

6. Constipation

Constipation may occur due to lack of appetite, inactivity, change in diet and intake of pain-killers.

Obstruction or blockage of the bowel is most often caused by cancer of the large bowel. It usually starts slowly with an occasional attack just like colic pain, in the abdomen. The pain is often accompanied by loud bowel sounds and swelling of the abdomen. The symptoms of complete bowel obstruction are colicky abdominal pain, nausea and vomiting.

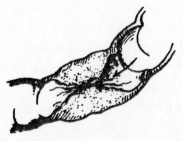

Constipation may become so complete that the patient is unable to pass even wind.

Natural Remedies: Constipation can be treated successfully by taking daily warm water enema. *The procedure for this treatment has been explained in chapter 9 on Natural Methods of Treatment.* This condition can also be overcome by liberal intake of fruits in the diet. Fruits very effective in curing constipation are grapes, pear, papaya and guava.

Spinach is another valuable remedy for constipation. Raw spinach contains the finest organic material for cleansing, reconstruction and regeneration of the intestinal tract. Raw spinach juice taken at the rate of half a litre daily can cure the most chronic cases of constipation within a few days.

7. Depression

Depression is very common in cancer. The older patients are especially prone to this disorder. They suffer from an acute sense of loss and inexplicable sadness, loss of energy and loss of interest.

Natural Remedies: As a rich source of magnesium, bananas have been found beneficial in the treatment of depression. Researches have shown that increased magnesium intake results in less anxiety and better sleep. Other rich sources of magnesium are nuts, beans and leafy green vegetables.

The use of apples is also considered valuable in depression. The various chemical substances present in this fruit, such as vitamin B1, phosphorus and potassium, help the synthesis of glutamic acid, which controls the wear and tear of the nerve cells. At least one apple should be eaten daily with milk and honey. This will act as a very effective nerve tonic and recharge the nerves with new energy and life.

8. Insomnia

Insomnia or sleeplessness is quite common in cancer patients. This may result from depression and stress and anxiety which are usually associated with cancer.

Natural Remedies: Lettuce is an effective remedy for overcoming sleeplessness as it contains a sleep-inducing substance known as 'lectucarium'. The juice of this plant has been likened in effect to the sedative action of opium without the accompanying excitement.

Milk is very valuable in insomnia. A glass of milk, sweetened with honey, should be taken every night before

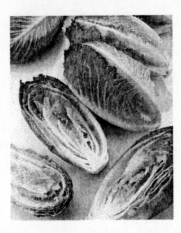

going to bed to treat this condition. It acts as a tonic and a tranquiliser. Massaging the milk over the soles of the feet has also been found to be effective.

9. Sore Mouth

Sore Mouth may result from drug reaction, vitamin deficiency, small ulcers, fungal infections and bacterial infections.

Natural Remedies: The treatment for sores in the mouth produced by drugs, is to keep the mouth hygienically clean. The patient should also gargle several times daily, with lemon juice mixed in water. This gargle can be prepared by mixing 20 ml. of lemon juice in 100 ml. of hot water.

A simple but effective home remedy for ulcers and infection in the mouth is frequent use of a mouth-wash containing a teaspoon each of salt and baking soda in a glass of warm water. This should be used every two to three hours to keep the mouth as clean as possible. The use of alum (*phitkari*) is also valuable in these conditions. The patient should gargle with alum diluted in hot water. Concentrated solution of alum may also be applied with the help of a swab on the ulcerated spots.

Other symptoms of cancer are blood in the sputum, motions and urine; changes in the menstrual periods, especially heavy and excessive bleeding between periods; changes in appearance, size and colour of moles which are present for a long time; abnormal delay in healing of any sore, particularly on the face; difficulty in passing urine; a persistent dry cough; indigestion occurring for the first time in later life; raised birth mark and tender swelling of the bone and the tissue.

The American Cancer Society has prescribed seven signs or danger signals in general, which may indicate the presence of cancer. These are a sore that does not heal, change in bowel or bladder habits, unusual bleeding or discharge, thickening or lump in breast or elsewhere, indigestion or difficulty in swallowing, obvious change in wart or mole and persistent and nagging cough or hoarseness.

Cancers have a latency period varying from five to forty years between the initial exposure to a carcinogen and the time the symptoms appear. In a large number of cases, either trivial symptoms are noted or there are none at all. One has therefore, to be vigilant to recognise the first sign of the disease.

CAUSES OF CANCER

3

There are numerous factors which play a role in the development of a cancer, but the prime cause of cancer is not known. Certain cancer-causing substances, known as carcinogens, however, increase the chances of getting the disease. About 80 per cent of cancers are caused by environmental factors. Many cancers are caused by habits, customs and usages.

Some well recognized and scientifically proven causes of cancer are mentioned herein:

1. Smoking

The most important cause of cancer is excessive smoking. This has been firmly established by various research studies conducted all over the world. These studies have shown that excessive smoking causes cancer of the lungs, stomach, respiratory organs, lips and mouth.

Approximately 40 per cent of male cancers in India are linked with tobacco, a known cancer-causing agent. The consumption of paan, betelnut, tobacco and slaked lime has been linked with cancer of the tongue, lips, mouth and throat. Cigarette and beedi smoking and hukka puffing are linked with lung and throat cancers.

2. Alcohol

Alcohol is injurious to health. Its excessive use can lead to development of cancer and many other serious diseases.

It can increase the risk of cancers of the upper and lower digestive tract, liver, prostate and breast. Those who consume excessive alcohol are particularly prone to colon cancer.

Smoking and drinking together makes matters worse. According to a study of European men by the International Agency for Research on Cancer in Lyon, France, the combination of heavy smoking and drinking can make persons 43 times more likely to develop throat cancer and 135 times more apt to get nasal cancer. Heavy beer drinking is especially linked to rectal cancer. Usually, the more alcohol consumed, the greater the risk of various cancers.

Moreover, new research suggests that drinking a lot of alcohol at one time can stimulate cancer to spread, by depressing the immune system. According to Gayle Page of the University of California at Los Angeles, even a few incidences of intoxication at feasts are considered sufficient to promote tumour progression. She says that in animals, the equivalent of four to five drinks in an hour, doubled the number of new lung tumours that had spread from the breast. Persons who are already suffering from cancer should be especially careful and avoid the consumption of alcohol completely.

3. Prolonged Irritation

It has been known for centuries that prolonged mechanical, physical and chemical irritation of the skin or mucous membranes can cause cancer. The edge of a broken tooth rubbing against the tongue, gall stones rubbing constantly against the gall-bladder, and smoking of short clay pipes used by labourers in Europe, have led to cancers of tongue, gallbladder and the lips respectively.

In the Godavari region of Andhra Pradesh, many men and women smoke locally rolled cigars (chutta) with the burning end inside the mouth. Some of these people are known to develop cancer of the mouth. Cancer below the umblicus, seen among Maharastrain men and women has been attributed to wearing of tight dhotis and sarees causing chronic irritation.

Excessive and continued drinking of very hot beverages may cause cancer of the throat and stomach. Prolonged irritation of the skin by chemicals or drugs may lead to skin cancer and continuous irritation of warts, pimples or slow healing sores may result in malignant tumours.

4. Drugs and Environmental Chemicals

The present era is full of chemical pollution all around. The air, water and foods, all contain thousands of man-made toxic chemicals. Most of them are potential carcinogens. According to Dr. Alfred Taylor of the biology institute of the University of Texas, even sodium fluoride in fluoridated water is linked to cancer growth. Several commonly used drugs are considered by many resarchers to be possible carcinogens.

Many widely-used pesticides are also definite carcinogens. Animal Studies commissioned by HEW and conducted by Bionetics Research Laboratories of Bethesda, Maryland, showed that more than half of all mice given oral doses of DDT developed tumours. In spite of mounting evidence that DDT is a proven carcinogen, it is widely used on food crops all over the world, including India.

5. Industrial Pollutants

Occupational exposure to industrial pollutants such as asbestos, nickel, tar and soot can lead to skin and lung cancers and leukaemia. Aromatic amines used in the manufacture of synthetic dyes cause cancer of urinary bladder. Radium and other radioactive elements produce cancer of the bone.

Workers in some branches of the dye industry develop

cancer of the bladder. The compounds found to be responsible are 2-naphthylamine and benzidine. Arsenites and arsenious oxide may produce cancer of the skin, if applied over a period of time.

Many persons working with X-rays, develop cancers of the skin and those exposed to radiation develop leukaemia. Ultraviolet radiation may, in certain circumstances, cause cancer of the skin.

6. High Protein Diet

Dr. Josef Issels, one of the foremost cancer specialist in the world and director of his world famous cancer clinic, says, "Excessive eating of meat and other cholesterol rich foods not only contributes to atherosclerosis and consequently, impaired blood circulation and diminished oxygenation of cells, but also increases the risk of tumour development". Research studies have shown that limiting the use of meat and animal fats, including butter, will reduce the risk of cancer.

Over-consumption of protein not only causes deficiencies of Vitamin B_6 B_3 and magnesium, but also a chronic pancreatic enzyme deficiency, which is considered one of the most important causes of cancer in countries with high protein consumption. It has been statistically demonstrated that countries with high animal protein consumption have a greater incidence of cancer and countries where the traditional diet is low in animal protein, even low in any kind of protein, have little or no cancer at all. Americans eat more protein than any other country in the world and they also lead the world in cancer statistics. Most leading cancer researchers and nutritionally-oriented doctors, such as Dr. Max Gerson, Dr. Werner Kollath and Dr. Alan H. Nittler, are convinced that overindulgence in protein and the body's inability to properly digest and utilize it, is one of the prime causes of cancer.

7. Over-eating

It is generally agreed that people usually eat more than their requirements. This leads to obesity, which is one of the most important cause of diseases of modern civilization and most degenerative diseases, including cancer. Studies on animals conducted by Dr. Issels indicate that those animals that were allowed to eat as much as they wished had 5.3 times more spontaneous cancer tumours than those animals that fasted every second day. During both the World Wars and immediately thereafter, when there was scarcity of food, cancer and other degenerative diseases virtually disappeared. The incidence of cancer again increased when food rationing was withdrawn. Even the National Cancer Institute in the United States acknowledges the relationship between over-eating and cancer.

For the same reasons, it has generally been observed that a high calorie diet and consequent increase in body weight beyond the optimum, increase the chances of developing cancer, especially in elderly men.

8. Nutritional Deficiencies

According to recent statistics from the U.S. Department of Agriculture and the U.S. Department of Health, Education and Welfare, about one half of all Americans suffer from various degrees of malnutrition and nutritional deficiencies. It has been shown in more than a hundred studies from around the world that almost any serious nutritional deficiency of one or more vitamins, minerals or other nutritive substances can lower the resistance to spontaneous cancer and increase the risk of contracting the disease. Thus, even a mild deficiency of Choline will produce cancer of the liver, Vitamin E deficiency increases the risk of contracting cancer and leukaemia, deficiencies of various B-Vitamins result in liver damage which leads to malignancies, serious deficiency of the mineral zinc may lead to cancer of the prostate, Vitamin A deficiency breaks down the body's defenses against most carcinogens and leads to tumour development, Magnesium deficiency is also linked to cancer development, as shown in studies conducted at the University of Montreal, in Egypt, and other places.

9. Exposure to Sun

Numerous studies have conclusively established that excessive and continuous exposure to the sun's ultraviolet rays can cause cancer of the skin in some people. Rimless eyeglasses, which concentrate the sun's reflections, are especially harmful and they can lead to skin cancer on the face.

10. Artificial Sex Hormone

A recent report of food and drug administration of the United State, shows that diethylstilbestrol, an artificial sex hormone widely used in food production, is a causative factor in cancer of the uterus, breast and other reproductive organs. This report is based on extensive research studies conducted in U.S.A. and many other countries. It has been established that 85 per cent of all meat in the United States contains dangerous residues of stilbestrol.

11. Hormone Imbalance

Cancer can also be caused by certain hormonal imbalances which if removed, can help control the disease. For instance, cancer of the prostate in men and that of the breast in women can be greatly relieved by the removal of the testes and ovaries respectively, in these patients, or by the removal of the adrenal glands which are a secondary source of sex hormones in both sexes. Besides this, administration of counter hormones like estrogen in males and androgen in females in such cases, also bring about remarkable improvement.

12. Saccharin

Saccharin, an artificial sweetener, which was discovered more than 100 years ago and has been widely used since then, can cause cancer. The Food and Drug Administration of the United State has recently removed it from its Generally Recognised As Safe (GRAS) list. Reliable animal tests conducted by an University of Wisconsin Research team, showed that saccharin causes cancer in the bladder and uterus. This artificial sweetener, however, is still being sold and used in U.S.A. and other countries. In the United States itself, over five million pounds of saccharin is used by the food industry each year.

13. Smog

Ozone, carbon monoxide, nitrogen dioxide and other photochemical pollutants in common smog have been implicated by many researchers as definite carcinogens. Smog now covers most of the advanced countries and no one can escape its carcinogenic effect. Carcinogenic chemicals present in smog cause cancer and many other health disorders, specially in the lungs and other respiratory organs.

14. Excessive X-rays

It has been scientifically established that excessive x-rays, which are used prophylactically or diagnostically by doctors, dentist and chiropractors, can cause cancer and leukaemia. Leukaemia in children, in later years, is often caused by pre-natal abdominal x-rays received by the mother during pregnancy.

15. Cadmium

Although beneficial in minute amounts, the trace element, cadmium, is extremely toxic in larger amounts. It is present in increasing amounts in our environment mostly from automobiles, phosphate fertilizers and various industries. It pollutes the soil and the water, and is taken up by plants, particularly by cereal grains. According to Dr. Lars Friberg of Sweden, wheat takes up ten times as much cadmium as rice. This trace element is concentrated in the liver of animals, which makes it a very dangerous food. It is also contained in shellfish to a dangerous level.

16. Rancid foods and Oils

Modern food processing and marketing have increased the risk of cancer. With the emphasis on long shelf-life, many foods are stale and rancid before they are consumed. Even natural, unprocessed health foods like wheat germ, wheat germ oil, sunflower seeds, sesame seeds and whole wheat flour sold in the market are stale. They are wonder foods if eaten absolutely fresh. Natural, unprocessed foods are highly perishable and they turn rancid within few days. Rancid foods are extremely dangerous. The vitamins, such as Vitamin E, A and F, for which we eat many of these foods, are completely destroyed in rancid foods. Besides, many harmful chemical substances, such as peroxides and others, are formed in the process of becoming rancid and these chemicals can cause cancer. This is also acknowledged by Dr. H. Anemueller of Germany, who is the foremost authority on rancid foods in the world. Fats when heated, especially vegetable fats, to a high temperature, become carcinogenic.

17. Sexually Transmitted Diseases

The incidence of cancer of the uterine cervix has increased in recent years, particularly among younger women. This has coincided with changing social patterns of greater sexual freedom and the use of oral contraceptives. This suggests that sexually transmissible diseases may cause this type of cancer. It is also observed that some cancers usually follow sexually transmitted diseases like syphilis and gonorrhoea.

18. Viruses

Some viruses can also cause cancer. Several cases of cancers in animals and birds have been attributed to viruses. Latest scientific studies have established that Leukaemia and Hodgkin's disease — a malignant disease of the lymphatic tissue, are associated with some kind of virus.

19. Chronic Depression in the Elderly

Chronic depression in the elderly can also lead to the development of cancer. According to a recent study conducted by Dr. Richard J.Havlik, of the National Institute of Aging in Bethesda, Maryland, and his associates, elderly persons who are chronically depressed for at least six years have 88 per cent higher risk of cancer than those who are not depressed. The authors of this study have noted that the previous researches found links between depression and cancer, mainly in smokers. But in this study, the "excess risk of cancer associated with chronic depression was consistent for most types of cancer and was not especially related to cigarette smokers".

20. Vaccinations

According to an eminent naturopath of India, K. Lakshmana Sarma, vaccinations can cause cancer. He observes that the substances introduced through vaccinations and inoculations "Combine with the molecules of the body-cells", and so alter their character in a profound and interesting manner. This re-arrangement of the molecules is of a more or less permanent character in many individuals, and in this case, persists for a considerable time. The very common use of vaccinations and inoculations in recent times, has a significant bearing upon the increase in the incidence of cancer.

Several European doctors also agree with this view. Dr. W.B. Clark of Indianapolis says, "Cancer was practically unknown until copox vaccination began to be introduced. I have had to do with at least 200 cases of cancer and I never saw a case of cancer in an unvaccinated person." Another doctor, Dr. E.J. Post of Berlmont, Michigan says, "I have removed cancers from vaccinated arms exactly where the poison was applied".

According to Medical Voodoo, in more than 100 years of vaccination, in England and Wales, cancer has increased by 92 per cent and the yearly rate of increase is now about 20 per cent of the total death rate in 1938. Dr. Wm. Lautie, late Medical Director of Metropolitan Cancer Hospital of London said "I am thoroughly convinced that persistent vaccination is an important contributing cause of cancer increase".

21. Aluminium

Aluminium is a powerful astringent with definite irritant qualities. Dr. H.W. Keens of London, England, in his recent publication titled Death in the (aluminium) Pot published by the C.W. Daniel Co., London, has come to the conclusion that aluminium cooking utensils play an important role in causing cancer. He says "After oxygen and silicon, aluminium is the most plentiful element and is indigenous to all soils..... It becomes toxic to organic tissues only when rendered soluble through its interactions with certain elements and compounds.... Soda, sulphur and ammonia appear to have the property of bringing aluminium out of its normal compounds and rendering it free and soluble to interact with other causative agents of some diseases of organic matter in the respect that it favours abnormal physiological functions".

22. Severe Emotional Stress

Personality traits play an important part in cancer development. Dr. Helen Flanders Dunbar claims that only certain types of people succumb to cancer. Popular health pioneer, J.I. Rodale, is of the opinion that happy people do not get cancer. Recent studies by such researchers as Dr. L.Leshan of the Institute of Applied Biology at New York University, Dr. Arthur Schmale, Jr. and Dr. Howard Iker of the University of Roschester Medical Center, and Dr. William Greene, Jr. of the University of Rochester Medical Center, all came up with findings that people with a lowered ability to deal with severe emotional conflicts and stresses, people with uncontrolled anxieties and worries, those with traumatic emotional experiences or losses are more pre-disposed to succumb to cancer.

23. Lowered Vitality

The primary and ultimate cause of cancer, however, is lowered vitality and a break down of the body's own defense mechanism against the physical, chemical, emotional and environmental stresses. This condition is brought about by an unnatural mode of living, over-feeding, over-excitement of the nerves through stimulants, or by medicaments for a long time. Many well-known biologists and naturopaths believe that a faulty diet is the root cause of cancer. Investigations indicate that the cancer incidence is in direct proportion to the amount of animal protein, particularly meat, in the diet.

It has been observed in the nutritional field for centuries, that people who live according to natural methods and follow natural laws in eating and living habits, do not get cancer. On the contrary, people who follow methods of modern nutrition on an increasing scale become prone to degenerative diseases, including cancer, in a relatively short time.

In later medical history, the best known cancer-free people were the Hunzas, who live on the slopes of the Himalayan mountains and who use only foods grown organically in their own country. They do not take imported foods. The same is true for the Ethiopians. They also have natural agriculture and simple living habits, which seems to prove that this type of agriculture keeps people free of cancer and most degenerative diseases.

DIET TO FIGHT CANCER 4

Diet is now considered a major factor in the prevention and treatment of cancer. According to the American National Cancer Institute, about one-third of all cancers are linked to diet. Thus, right choices of foods can help prevent a majority of new cancer cases and deaths from cancer.

Faulty Diet-Basic Cause of Cancer

Many great pioneers, biological and naturopathic doctors, as well as those practising at present, notably Dr. Bircher-Benner, Dr. Duncan Bulkley, A. Vogel, Max Gerson, Dr. Kristine Nolfi, Dr. Ragnar Berg, Dr. Are Waeland, Dr. Werner Zabel, Dr. J.H. Tilden, and Dr. Alice Chase, believe that faulty diet can be a basic cause of cancer.

Based on their own extensive practice and by studying the eating habits of cancer-free natives and people around the world, their conclusions emphatically pointed to the fact that, in addition to well-known environmental carcinogens, such as smoking, chemical poisons in foods and environment and other factors, the cancer incidence is in direct propotion to the amount of animal proteins, particularly meat, in the diet.

Cancer usually develops over a long period. Latest research shows that what one eats may interfere with the cancer process at many stages, from conception to growth and spread of the cancer. Foods can block the chemical activation, which normally initiates cancer. Antioxidants, including vitamins, can eradicate carcinogens and can even repair some of the cellular damage caused by them. Cancers, which are in the process of growth, can also be prevented from spreading further by foods. Even in advanced cases, the right food can prolong the patient's life.

Fruits and Vegetables-Antidote to Cancer

Researches conducted in ascertaining links between diet and cancer since 1970, have now conclusively proved that fruits and vegetables can serve as antidotes to cancer. According to Dr. Peter Greenwald, Director of the Division of Cancer Prevention and control at the American National Cancer Institute, "The more fruits and vegetables people eat, the less likely they are to get cancer, from colon and stomach cancer to breast and even lung cancer. For many cancers, persons with high fruit and vegetable intake have about half the risk of people with low intake."

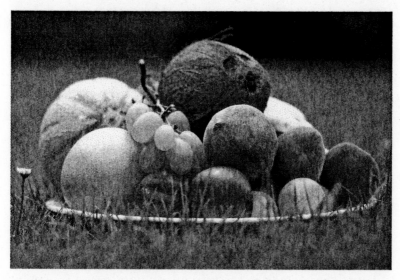

Some studies indicate that eating fruits twice a day cuts the risk of lung cancer by 75 per cent, even in smokers. The normal servings of fruits and vegetables are two fruits and three vegetables a day. Adding more fruits and vegetables to these servings can reduce the risk of cancer. One serving means 100-115g of cooked or chopped raw fruit or vegetables, 70-85g of raw leafy vegetables, one medium piece of fruit, or 170 ml of fruit juice or vegetable juice.

Sulphur rich Vegetables —— Reduce Risk of Cancer

A survey of dietary habits in China from 1973-1984 found, among other things, that people who ate more sulphur-rich vegetables like cabbage, cauliflower, garlic and onions had the lowest risks of cancer, in general.

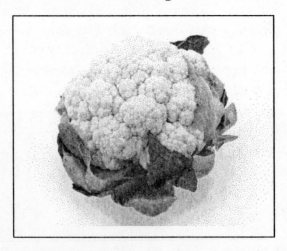

Persons who avoid raw fruits and vegetables are more prone to stomach cancer. Several studies have found an array of fruits and raw vegetables to be so protective, that anyone worried about stomach cancer should simply increase the intake of raw vegetable and fruit salads. If a person does not consume raw foods daily, his risk of stomach cancer doubles or even triples, according to studies conducted in Japan, England and Poland. Raw vegetables of various types are powerful anti-stomach cancer foods, according to extensive research. Especially protective are raw celery, cucumbers, carrots, green peppers, tomatoes, onions and lettuce.

Anti-cancer Diet

According to the leading biological cancer specialists in Europe viz, Zabel, Issels, Kollath, Meyer, Lampert, Kuhl and Warburg there is, indeed, such a thing as an anti-cancer diet- a diet that can help prevent cancer, as well as help the body to cure it.

Dr. Issels advises the following anti-cancer diet to help the body prevent cancer, or to assist the body's healing mechanism, when cancer has already developed:

1. diet must consist exclusively of organically grown foods, which are free from carcinogenic chemicals, such as toxic additives, insecticide residues, preservatives and other man-made chemicals.
2. most foods must be eaten in their natural, raw state, especially fresh fruits and raw vegetable salad.
3. nuts should form a part of the daily diet. The best nuts are almonds and walnuts.
4. the diet should include generous amounts of fermented (lactic acid) foods, such as naturally fermented grains and fermented juices. According to Dr. Johannes Kuhl, the originator of the lactic acid fermentation diet for cancer, 50 to 75 per cent of the daily diet should be made up of lactic acid fermented foods.
5. the diet should include moderate amount of easily-digested proteins. These should comprise mostly vegetable origin, foods, such as green leafy vegetables, potatoes, sprouted seeds and grains, nuts, and raw, unheated, home-made cottage cheese from high quality unpasterised milk.

6. all other animal proteins like meat, fowl, eggs or fish should be completely eliminated from the diet.

7. milk and milk products should be taken mostly in fermented and soured forms. The best forms of soured milks are acidophilus milk, natural buttermilk and home-made soured milk, preferably made from goat's milk. Goat's milk is better than cow's milk. Raw goat's milk of high quality, contains anti-cancer and antiarthritis factors.

8. avoid saturated, and cholestrol-rich animal fats, including butter. These should be replaced with a moderate amount of genuine, cold-pressed vegetable oils, especially sunflower seed oil, flaxseed oil, soya bean oil and safflower oil. Oils should never be heated.

9. eliminate from the diet, all processed and denatured foods, especially all refined carbohydrates, such as white flour and white sugar, and all foods made from them.

At least three-fourth of the food consumed should consist of all kinds of fruits, mostly fresh; freshly prepared juices from fruits such as orange, grapefruit, grapes, apple and pineapple; fruit salads; mashed bananas, raw grated apples, and apple sauce; raw or freshly-prepared steamed or lightly-cooked vegetables such as carrots, cabbage, cauliflower, celery, tomato, onion and baked potatoes; and whole grain cereals and milk and milk products like curd, butter milk and cottage cheese.

The treatment of cancer thus consists of a complete change in diet, besides total elimination of all environmental sources of carcinogens. As a first step, the patient should cleanse the system by thoroughly relieving constipation and making all the organs of elimination active. Warm-water enema should be used daily to cleanse the bowels.

Raw Juices for cleansing the System

For the first four or five days, the patient should take fresh fruits or vegetable juices, diluted with water on a 50:50 basis, every two hours from 8 a.m. to 8 p.m.. The fruits and vegetables which can be used for juicing are apple, pineapple, grapes, grapefruit, orange, peach, pear, papaya, carrot, cabbage, celery and beet-root. Beet juice will be especially beneficial. Other beneficial juices are those extracted from carrot, grapes and generally, all dark coloured juices. The purpose of juice fasting is to normalize all the vital body processes, revitalize the liver and other cleansing organs. Juice fasting will cleanse the whole body of accumulated toxins, restore the digestive and assimilative functions of the stomach and intestinal tract, and in general, increase the body's protective and healing capacity. After the short juice fast, the patient may adopt an exclusive diet of fresh fruits for further five days. In this regime, he should take three meals a day of fresh juicy fruits like apple, pineapple, orange, grapes and grapefruit, at five-hourly intervals. Thereafter, he may gradually embark upon a well-balanced, nourishing, alkaline-based diet.

The diet should consist of 100 per cent natural foods, with emphasis on fresh fruits and raw vegetables, particularly carrots, green leafy vegetables, cabbage, onion, garlic, cucumber, beet and tomatoes. A minimum requirement of high quality protein, mostly from vegetable sources such as almonds, millet, sprouted seeds and grains, may be added to this diet. The short juice fast, followed by an exclusive diet of fresh fruits, may be repeated at regular intervals till this condition improves.

The patient should avoid tea, coffee, cocoa, white flour, white sugar and all products made with white flour and sugar. He should also avoid flesh foods of all kinds, eggs, cheese, dairy butter, strong condiments, pickles, alcohol and smoking. Salt should be used sparingly.

Precautions for Cooking Vegetables

Certain precautions are necessary while cooking vegetables for use by cancer patients. All vegetables must be cooked over a low flame, without addition of water. This will preserve the natural flavor of the vegetables and will make them easily digestible. Valuable minerals are lost by excessive heat – as the cells burst, minerals lose their colloidal composition and are thus not absorbed easily. An asbestos mat may be used to prevent burning. Tomatoes may be placed at the bottom of the pan to make available more fluid. This also improves flavor in some cases. Spinach water however, should be discarded as it contains too much oxalic acid. Red beet should be cooked like potatoes, with their peel in water. All vegetables must be thoroughly washed and cleaned. Peeling or scraping of vegetable should be avoided as important mineral salts and vitamins are deposited directly under the skin. The cooking pot should be closed tightly, to prevent escape of steam.

Pressure cookers should not be used for cooking of vegetable, nor saucepans or other utensils of aluminium. Stainless steel, glass, enamel, earthenware and cast iron utensils may be used.

FOODS THAT PREVENT AND CONTROL CANCER

Cancer progresses slowly. It starts with the "Initiation" of a single cell by cancer-causing substances. According to John D. Poter, M.D., of the University of Minnesota, foods and food compounds can interfere with this cancer process at about ten stages of development. Food compounds can prevent activation of cancer-causing agents. They can block the mutation of a cell's genetic material. They can stimulate enzymes in the body, which remove cancer-causing chemicals out of the body.

These compounds can prevent cancer-causing oncogens from becoming active. They can combat bacteria which cause stomach cancer. They can manipulate hormones and neutralize toxic agents that promote cancer. These compounds can reduce the ability of cancerous cells to proliferate and form tumours. They can even help prevent cancer cells from spreading to establish new cancers. Fruits and vegetables have high concentration of anticancer compounds.

There are certain foods, which can serve the purpose of chemotherapy after the development of cancer. The chemicals contained in these foods have chemotherapeutic powers to fight cancer by retarding tumour growth, spread and recurrence. They can even attack malignancy by destroying cancer cells. Foods with such chemical compounds can be used as supportive therapy to modern medical cancer treatments.

Foods which possess major anti-cancer activities are beet,

cabbage and other cruciferous vegetables, carrot, citrus fruits (grapefruit, lemon, lime and orange), curd, garlic, green vegetables, liquorice, milk, olive-oil, rice (brown), soya beans, tomato, watermelon, wheat bran and some other foods. The use of these foods for the prevention and controlling of various kinds of cancer are discussed herein.

Beet

The juice of red beet is considered beneficial in the prevention and treatment of cancer. It is one of the best

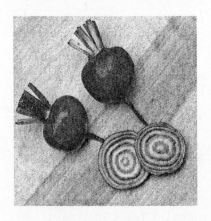

vegetable juices and a rich source of natural sugar. It contains sodium, potassium, phosphorus, calcium, sulphur, chlorine, iodine, iron, copper, vitamin B_1, B_2, niacin, B_6, C and P. This juice stimulates the liver and its detoxifying activity. Half a glass of this juice can be taken three times daily. Lactic acid a well balanced beet juice will markedly increase the oxygenation of the body cells. It would be advisable to extract juice both, from the root and top.

Cabbage and other Cruciferous Vegetables

Cabbage and other cruciferous vegetables like cauliflower and Brussel sprouts are one of the most important foods which may help immunize against breast cancer by managing oestrogen, a known promoter of this type of cancer. These vegetables quickly remove oestrogen from the body by speeding up the metabolism of oestrogen and burning up the hormone so that less of it is available to feed cancer. This has been revealed by the research studies conducted by Dr. Jon Michnovicz and his colleagues at the Institute of Hormone Research, in New York city. These studies indicate that specific indoles in these cruciferous vegetables accelerate a process in which the body deactivates or disposes off the type of oestrogen that can promote breast cancer.

In tests on women and men, the cabbage compound "turned up" the oestrogen-deactivation process by about 50 per cent, says Dr. Michnovicz. The test dose, exceeded what people would normally eat: a daily 500 milligrams of indole-3-carbinol, the amount in about 400g of raw cabbage, but eating less would also burn up oestrogen to a lesser degree. It's known that women with elevated oestrogen metabolism have lower risks of hormone-dependent cancers, such as breast, uterine and endometrial cancer, says Dr. Michnovicz.

The use of cabbage in its raw form has also been found valuable in preventing colon cancer, according to Dr. Jim Duke at the U.S. Department of Agriculture, who had a family history of colon cancer. Dr. Duke says his colon polyps diminished dramatically after he ate raw cabbage every other

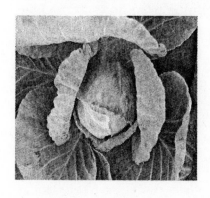

day. According to another expert, Dr. Greenwald, other fibre-rich vegetables can also reduce the risk of colon cancer. His analysis of 37 studies conducted in the past 20 years, showed that eating high-fibre foods, including vegetables, cut the chances of colon cancer by 40 per cent.

Carrot

This vegetable is one of the richest sources of beta carotene. It has been found valuable in preventing lung cancer.

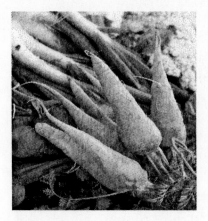

Beta carotene, it may be mentioned, is an orange pigment isolated from carrots more than 150 years ago. It acts as an antidote to lung cancer. A recent study at the State University of New York at Buffalo, shows that eating beta carotene-rich vegetables more than once a week dramatically reduced chances of lung cancer when compared with people who do not eat such vegetables. Munching a single raw carrot at least twice a week reduces the risk of lung cancer by 60 per cent. The anti-cancer power of beta carotene comes from both its antioxidant capabilities and its ability to enhance immunological defenses, which are very important in preventing and fighting cancer.

Citrus Fruits

Citrus fruits like grapefruit, lemon, lime and orange

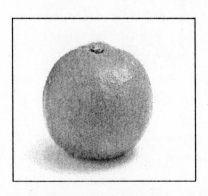

possess powerful anti-cancer properties. Toxicologist Herbert Pierson, Ph.D., a diet and cancer expert, formally with the American National Cancer institute, considers citrus fruits a total anti-cancer package, as they possess every class of natural substances like carotenoids, flavonoids, terpenes, lemonades and coumarins, which individually, have neutralized powerful chemical carcinogens in animals. One analysis found that citrus fruits possess 58 known anti-cancer chemicals, more than any other food. Dr. Pierson further says: "The beauty of citrus is that several classes of phytochemicals are highly likely to act more powerfully... as a natural mixture than when they appear separately." In other words, whole citrus fruits are marvellous combinations of anticancer compounds. One such anti-cancer compound is glutathione.

Whole oranges contain high concentrations of this tested disease-antagonist. However, when extracted, the juice tends to lose glutathione concentrations. Oranges, of all foods, are also the richest source of glucarate, another cancer-inhibitor. Some experts have linked the wide-spread use of citrus fruits with the dramatic decline of stomach cancer in the United States.

Curd

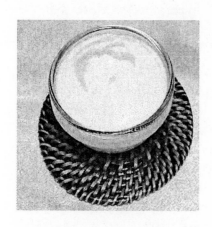

Curd or yogurt is a potential preventive against colon cancer. It is a rich source of vitamin D and calcium, both of which are highly beneficial in preventing cancer. Research studies show that Lactobacillus acidophilus helps suppress enzyme activity needed to convert otherwise harmless substances into cancer-causing chemicals in the colon. This has been brought out in the studies conducted by leading researchers Barry R. Goldin and Sherwood L. Gorbach at the New England Medical Centre. For a month, volunteers drank two glasses of plain milk everyday, thereafter, they switched to acidophilus milk. When enzyme activity was measured in the subject's colon, it was found that drinking acidophilus milk helped dangerous enzyme activity to drop by 40-80 per cent. This means certain carcinogenic activity in the colon was dramatically suppressed.

Garlic

Garlic is an ancient remedy for cancer. Even the father

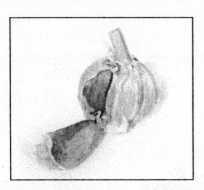

of medicine, Hippocrates prescribed garlic for this disease more than two thousand years ago. It was, however, only in the twentieth century that scientists discovered the anti-cancer properties of garlic. The use of garlic has been found especially valuable in preventing stomach, lung and liver cancers. More than 30 different enemies of carcinogens have been identified in garlic and onions. Such compounds include diallyl sulphide, quercetin and ajoene. In animals, they block the most terrifying cancer-causing agents such as nitrosamines and aflatoxin, linked specifically to stomach, lung and liver cancer. In experiments, feeding garlic to animals consistently blocked cancer. Garlic also helps strengthen that part of the immune system, which directly fights tumours. It should thus form part of the diet of those who are having cancer or at risk of getting it. Various studies conducted in China, Italy and the United States during the last ten years, have conclusively proved the protective role of garlic in the diet, which can fight cancer effectively.

A five-year Designer Foods Program launched by the National Cancer Institute in U.S.A. in 1991, examined foods which were likely to prevent cancer, based on either traditional medicine or recent epidemiological studies. Among the foods selected were garlic, citrus fruit, linseed, liquorice root, and members of the parsley family. The researchers tried to ascertain the constituents in these foods which could help prevent the formation of cancer cells. According to Herbert F. Pierson, director of this program, garlic is the food with the greatest power to prevent cancer.

In 1994, research studies were conducted at the University of Minnesota to examine the relationship of diet and colon cancer in a large number of women from Iowa. These studies provided stronger scientific evidence than before, about the value of garlic in preventing colon cancer.

Michael Wargovich, at the Houston's M.D. Anderson Cancer Center, a leading researcher on garlic, gave some mice purified diallyl sulphide from garlic, and others, plain mice food, followed by powerful carcinogens. Mice fed on the garlic substances had 75 per cent less colon tumours. More impressive, when given agents that cause oesophageal cancer in mice, not a single one getting the diallyl sulphide came down with cancer! Similarly, John Milner, head of nutrition at Penn State university, succeeded in blocking 70 per cent of breast tumours in mice by feeding them fresh garlic. Studies on humans show that those who eat more onions and garlic are less prone to various cancers.

Garlic seems to prevent cells turning cancerous by increasing the body's natural mechanisms for removing toxic substances. The liver eliminates toxic chemicals and other substances from the body, and garlic protects the liver itself from damage. Garlic also has a deep effect on liver detoxification enzymes, which break down toxic substances and render them harmless. Garlic's many sulphur-rich compounds appear to be responsible for this effect. Sulphur makes up about one per cent of garlic by weight, and dozens of sulphur containing compounds are present in it, especially after it has been chopped or crushed. At the cell level, these sulphur compounds bind to sensitive areas in the cell's genetic machinery. By blocking those sites, the compounds appear to prevent cancer causing chemicals from doing their damage to the cell.

Garlic also protects against radiation-induced cancer. A certain level of radiation from the sun is normal in the atmosphere. This radiation puts the people who spend considerable time in the sun at great risk for skin cancer. Other sources of radiation in the atmosphere are, pollution from energy or weapons production. Eating garlic liberally can help prevent cancer caused by radiation from all these sources.

Green Vegetables

Green vegetables, especially green leafy vegetables exhibit unusual wide anti-cancer powers. A recent Italian study showed a powerful protection from the frequent consumption of green vegetables against the risk of most cancers. Green vegetables such as spinach, fenugreek, dark green lettuce and broccoli, are full of many different antioxidants, including beta carotene and folic acid, as well as lutein – a little-known antioxidant. Some scientists believe that lutein may even be

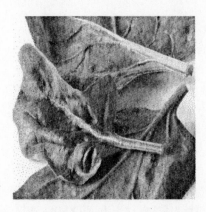 as powerful as beta carotene in blocking cancer. Green leafy vegetables are rich in lutein. Darkest green vegetables should be chosen to detive maximum carotenoids and other anticancer agents. According to Frederick Khachik, Ph.D., a research scientist at the Department of Agriculture, "The darker green they are the

most cancer preventing carotenoids they have". He also says lutein and other carotenoids are not lost during cooking or freezing, although heat exercises harmful effects on more fragile antioxidants, including vitamin C and glutathione.

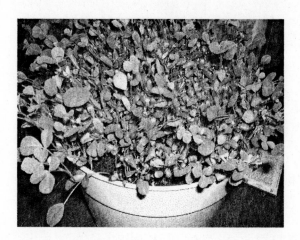

Liquorice

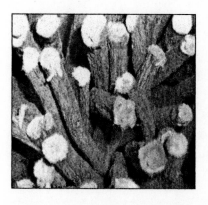

Liquorice, a popular spice and a flavouring agent, is credited with the properties of foods which not only help prevent cancer but also retard its spread. Triterpenoids contained in liquorice may block quick-growing cancer cells and cause some pre-cancerous cells to return to normal growth. This spice can be used either in the form of powder, decoction or infusion. The preparation can be taken mixed with honey.

Milk

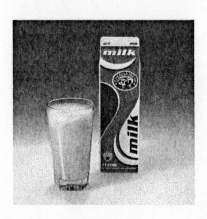

Milk, as a rich source of vitamin D and calcium, is an important food which can reduce the risk of colon cancer. Both these nutrients supress cancer in a powerful way. According to Dr. Cedric Garland, director of the Cancer Centre at the University of California at San Diego, blood levels of vitamin D can predict the risk of colon cancer. He examined 25,620 blood samples collected in Maryland in 1974, for vitamin D content and then he compared colon cancer rates over the next eight years. His conclusion was that those with high blood levels of vitamin D were 70 per cent less likely to develop colon cancer than those with low levels.

According to several studies, it appears that calcium suppresses harmful physiological factors leading to colon cancer. Dr. Cedric Garland has noted that men who drank a couple of glasses of milk daily over a 20 year period were only one-third as prone to developing colon cancer as non-milk drinkers. Dr. Garland estimates that 1,200-1,400mg of calcium per day might prevent 65-75 per cent of colon cancers. One reason is that calcium can suppress the proliferation of surface cells on the inner lining of the colon, thereby preventing the rapid cell growth which is a sign of developing cancer.

Olive Oil

Eating too much fat has been linked with breast cancer. This has been adequately proved by a research study of 750

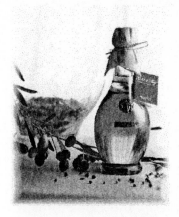

Italian women. It was found in this study that the women who eat the most saturated fats have triple the risk of breast cancer as compared to those eating the least. Eating too much fat can influence the spread and virulence of an existing breast cancer, its recurrence and survival chances. Some researches show that the more saturated animal fat in your diet, the greater the odds of auxillary lymph node involvement or spread of the cancer, and the more total fat in a diet, the greater the chances of dying from breast cancer. Monounsaturated fat, the type predominant in olive oil, is however, not cancer a culprit. In fact, new evidence suggests that olive-oil-type fat can help counteract cancer. Mediterranean women who eat lots of olive oil have low rates of breast cancer, as do Japanese women who eat lots of fish oils but little animal fat.

Rice

Rice possesses anti-cancer activity. Like other seeds, it contains anti-cancer protease inhibitors. The use of brown rice, is especially helpful in preventing cancer.

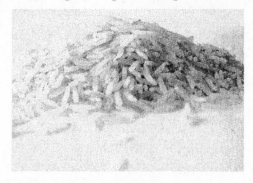

Soya-beans

This vegetable contains compounds which can manipulate oestrogen and also directly inhibit the growth of cancerous cells, thereby reducing the risk of breast cancer in women of all ages, according to Stephen Barnes, Ph.D., associate professor of pharmacology and biochemistry at the University of Alabama. One soya-bean compound, phytoestrogens is quite similar chemically, to the drug tamoxifen, which is given to certain women to help prevent breast cancer and its spread. Soya-bean also helps to block the growth of cancer cells in another way not related to oestrogen. Studies in cells have found that soyabean substances, for some unknown reasons, can entirely halt the growth of cancerous cells even though they do not have any oestrogen receptors to block, according to Dr. Barnes. That means these soya-bean compounds fight cancer in at least two separate ways, he says.

Tomato

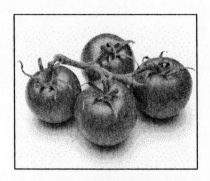

Tomato is regarded as an anti-cancer drug. Lycopene that gives it its colour, is the main ingredient which helps prevent cancer. A research study conducted by Dr. Helmut Sies of Germany has found that lycopene is twice as powerful as beta carotene at "quenching singlet oxygen," a rampaging toxic oxygen molecule that can trigger cancer in cells. Tomatoes are the major source of lycopene in the food supply, and that includes all types of tomato products, such as cooked tomatoes, canned tomatoes and sauces, tomato paste and ketchup.

Watermelon

This fruit being highly concentrated in lycopene, is also regarded as an anti-cancer food, which can help prevent cancer.

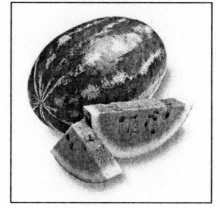

Wheat-bran

One way to reduce the chances of breast cancer is to curtail oestrogen levels in the blood. This can be achieved by taking wheat-bran cereals. Wheat-bran has specific properties to lower dramatically, the circulating levels of cancer-promoting oestrogen in the blood. This was found in a research study by David P. Rose, M.D., of the American Health Foundation in New York. In this study, some women were made to eat three to four high-fibre muffins a day made with either oat-bran, corn-bran or what-bran. That doubled their fibre intake from about 15g to 30g. After a month, there was a little difference in their blood oestrogen levels, but after two months, oestrogen levels had come down by about 17 per cent in the women eating wheat-bran. Oestrogen levels did not change in eaters of oat-bran or corn-bran muffins.

However, all type of brans, including wheat-bran are rich sources of fibre and can help reduce the risk of colon cancer. Studies consistently show that fibre-rich foods generally prevent colon cancer. Some specific foods, however, have shown outstanding powers in this regard. Wheat-bran has the best reputation as a powerful colon cancer fighter.

Other Foods

Certain other foods have also been found to contain anti-cancer activities and are thus valuable, in preventing and controlling cancer. These include cucumber, flax seeds, ginger, mints, oats, green peppers, potato, turmeric and whole wheat.

HARMFUL FOODS THAT PROMOTE CANCER

There are certain foods which help in promoting cancer and aggravate it, if it has already developed. These foods are fats, flesh foods and sugar. The harmful effects of these foods are described herein.

Coffee

Most of the coffee's pharmacological impact comes from its high concentration of caffeine, a psychoactive drug of great power, and the most active alkoloid principle in it. This is an addictive drug similar to cocaine in as much as it stimulates the central nervous system. These effects are short-lived, but it has been observed that they lead to withdrawal symptoms of irritability, lethargy, headaches and anxiety. This shows that it is a strong enough drug to constitute a potential health hazard.

Sir Robert Hutchison, an eminent nutritionist, found about 100 mg. of caffeine and 200 mg. of tannin in a cupful of coffee, made by infusing 60 g. in 450 ml. of water.

Research studies have shown that coffee drinking has potential health hazards. They have linked it to several serious diseases including cancer.

The harmful effects of coffee have been particularly observed on the gall bladder. It can stimulate the gall bladder to bring about gall bladder attacks. This may result in gallstone and ultimately gall bladder cancer. Bruce R. Douglas and colleagues at the University Hospital in Leiden, Netherlands, discovered in a test of healthy normal men and women, that drinking as little as 115 ml. of decaffeinated coffee stimulated gall bladder contractions. The researchers advise people prone to gallstones to avoid all types of coffee.

Fat

Scientific studies show that people with higher rates of cancer, consume excessive animal fat in their daily diet. Additionally, widely used omega-6 polyunsaturated fats, such as corn oil, are potential cancer threaths. For instance, feeding animals corn oil greatly increases cancer rates in those exposed to carcinogens.

Fat increases the risk of cancer in a variety of ways. It acts as a fuel to promote tumour growth. If fat is not used, cancer-prone cells might remain relatively inactive. Fat also stimulates bile acids in the colon that can help drive cells towards cancer. Additionally, eating too much fat, both animal and omega-6 vegetable oils, can depress the immune system's tumour surveillance mechanism. This has been proved by the studies conducted at the American Health Foundation and St. Luke's-Roosevelt Hospital Center, in New York.

Flesh Foods

Racial groups and nations whose diet contains less meat, show less cancer incidence than groups consuming high-meat diets. Hospital records show that Seventh Day Adventists, Mormons and Navajo Indians, who eat little or no meat, suffer far less from cancer than the average meat-eating Americans. Recently, a link between excessive meat-eating and cancer has been explained by Dr. Willard J. Visek, research scientist at Cornell University. Dr. Visek says that the high-protein diet of Americans is linked to the high incidence of cancer in the U.S. The villian, according to Dr. Visek, is ammonia, the carcinogenic by-product of meat digestion. Of all meats, pork is especially harmful. It has been noted that in places where pork is the principle diet, cancer seems to be most prevalent.

Our actual daily protein requirement is only between 20 and 30 grams, as shown by numerous studies around the world. Protein eaten in excess above the actual need, cannot be properly digested or utilized and acts in the body as a poison and carcinogen. In addition, over consumption of protein, taxes the pancreas and causes chronic deficiency of pancreatic enzymes, which are required for proper protein metabolism.

Moreover, flesh is often a carrier of disease germs. Diseases of many kinds are on the increase in animals, making flesh foods more and more unsafe. People are continually eating flesh that may contain tuberculosis and cancerous germs. Often animals are taken to the market and sold for food when they are so diseased that their owners do not wish to keep them any longer.

Excessive Salt

Many nutritionists believe that salt is too freely used in the ordinary diet and, could be one of the main causes of cancer. Most cancer patient are therefore, prescribed salt-free diets. It is claimed that salt is often responsible for excessive hydrochloric acid in the stomach. This burns and injures the tissues and leads to stomach ulcers, which may even develop into cancer. The Crile clinic in Cleveland insists on salt-free diets for patients suffering from stomach ulcers. The liberal intake of salt often nullifies the beneficial effects of foods such as celery, cucumbers, greens and spinach.

World Health Organization (WHO), reported from Japan that it has been statistically demonstrated that the frequency of cancer of the stomach in Japan, is definitely related to the quantity of salt consumed by the natives. The more salt in the diet, the more stomach cancer.

Sugar

Sugar is also considered harmful and its excessive consumption can lead to the development of cancer. Recently, a Nobel Prize winner of the University of Pennsylvania Medical School, Dr. Otto Meyerhoff, spoke of the evidence connecting the excessive consumption of sugar with cancer by calling attention to "the appetite of tumours for sugar." He suggested that the growth of cancerous tissue might possibly be stopped if biochemists could find a way of curing this appetite.

VITAMINS THAT FIGHT CANCER

Vitamins are powerful substances, which can help to block cancer. Recent research has shown that certain vitamins can be successfully employed in the fight against this disease and that they can increase the life expectancy of some terminal cancer patients.

Vitamin C

Vitamin C heads the list of vitamins found beneficial in the prevention and treatment of cancer. It is the most potent anti-toxin known. It can effectively neutralize or minimize the damaging effect of most chemical carcinogens in foods and the environment and, thus, be of great value in cancer prevention programs, as well as, in the treatment of cancer. It can be taken in large doses of 5,000 mg. or more a day.

Vitamin C can block the transformation of amines and nitrite into nitrosamines which are deadly carcinogens that can cause all types of cancer. It helps neutralize free radical cancer-causing agents in cell membranes thereby preventing the first step in cancer. It also helps regulate immunity and thus prevents transformation of healthy cells into cancerous cells. In experiments with animals, it has been found that this vitamin suppresses the growth and virulence of tumours.

According to recent Swedish studies, vitamin C in large doses can be an effective prophylactic agent against cancer. Noted Japanese scientist, Dr. Fukunir Mirishige and his colleagues have recently found that a mixture of vitamin C and copper compound has lethal effects on cancer.

There is growing evidence that many cancers are caused by viruses. Since vitamin C appears to nullify the damage done by viruses, this nutrient may prove to be particularly important. All types of cancer cause severe stress. This increases the need for vitamin C to a very large extent. Most cancer patients show symptoms of bruising, bleeding gums, and often, hemorrhaging, which is characteristic of a deficiency of vitamin C. It has been found that if a patient who cannot be operated, is given 4,000 to 6,000mg of vitamin C daily, it would inhibit the growth of cancer and in some cases, it may even retard its progress.

The main food sources of Vitamin C are citrus fruits and vegetables. Among fruits, Indian gooseberry, guava, lime, lemon, orange and papaya are the most valuable sources of this vitamin. Root vegetables and potatoes contain smaller amounts of these vitamins. Cereals and pulses do not contain vitamin C in the dry state. Nuts, if soaked in water for about 48 hours and allowed to germinate, form a good source of Vitamin C.

Vitamin A

Beta-Carotene, an orange pigment and a precursor of vitamin A has been linked with preventing cancer. It improves the functioning of the immune system and helps eliminate oxygen-type free radicals. It has been noted that cancer patients often have low blood levels of beta-carotene. In a study, beta-carotene levels in the blood of lung cancer patients was found to be one-third lower than that in healthy individuals. Similarly, according to a recent British study, it was found that men with the most beta-carotene in their blood were 60 per cent as likely to develop cancer, especially lung cancer, as those with the lowest blood beta-carotene.

According to several studies, vitamin A exerts an inhibiting effect on carcinogenesis. It is one of the most important aids in the body's defense system to fight and prevent cancer. Dr. Leonida Santamaria and his colleagues at the University of Pavis in Italy, have uncovered preliminary evidence suggesting that beta-carotene may actually inhibit skin cancer by helping the body thwart the cancer-causing process, known as oxidation. This vitamin can be taken in large doses upto 1,50,000 units a day in the treatment of cancer.

The main food sources of Beta Carotene are dark orange and dark green leafy vegetables – sweet potatoes, carrots, dried apricots, lady's finger, spinach and pumpkin. Other good sources of this vitamin are grapefuit, mangoes, lettuce and broccoli. The darker orange or green the fruit or vegetable, the more beta carotene it contains.

Vitamin B-complex

Many scientists believe that chronic oxygen deficiency in cells leads to the formation of cancer cells. Vitamin B increases the body's resistance to oxygen deficiency. In some experiments with animals, when they were given azo dyes deficient in Riboflavin or vitamin B_2, they died of cancer. However, when they were given adequate amounts of this vitamin, it prevented the development of cancers.

In some other studies, animals given dye-fed rats deficient in vitamin B_2, developed cancer of the lymph glands or liver. However when they were given the vitamin after the cancers were growing, it remarkably delayed further development of the disease. In some other experiments, several other B vitamins were found to exert a protective influence against many types of malignancies produced by various other means. Thus, cancers develop quickly when the diet is deficient in Pyridoxine or vitamins B_6, but excessive amounts cause vitamin B_2 to be excreted, thereby increasing cancer growth. Similarly, an excess of vitamin B_2, by inducing a deficiency of vitamin B_6, has caused tumours to grow more rapidly. It therefore, appears advisable that all B-vitamin supplements should contain the same amounts of vitamins B_2 and B_6.

Natural, high potency Vitamin B-Complex is considered important for the prevention of cirrhosis of the liver, which often leads to cancer. The incidence of cancer in a liver that has been affected by cirrhosis, is 60 times greater than in a normal liver. Studies also show that B-Vitamin deficient diets lead to a higher incidence of primary liver cancer as compared B-vitamin rich diets.

Dr. Otto Warburg, Nobel Prize winner and director of the Max plank institute for Cell Physiology in Berlin, and one of the leading cancer experts in the world, says that the primary cause of cancer is the lack of one or more of three B-Vitamins, namely riboflavin, niacin and pantothenic acid, in tissues subjected to carcinogens. Dr. Warburg says that a plentiful supply of these three vitamins in the diet is the best possible protection against cancer.

Food rich in riboflavin or B_2 are green vegetables such as turnip greens, beet, radish leaves, colocasia and carrot leaves and fruits such as papaya, raisins, custard apple and apricot. Other good sources of this vitamin are almonds, walnuts, pistachionuts, and mustard seeds. Vegetarian food sources of Niacin or B_3 are rice bran, rice, wheat, groundnuts, sunflower seeds and almonds and green vegetables like turnip and beet greens, the leaves of carrots, colocaisa, and celery. Good vegetarian food sources of pantothenic acid or B_5 are yeast, peanuts, mushrooms, split peas, soya-beans and soya-bean flour.

Vitamin E

Research studies have also shown that vitamin E may be

especially valuable in cancer prevention. In malignancy-induced animals, when vitamin E was administered in varying degrees, it was found that those who were given the most of this vitamin were fewest, smallest and slowest in developing malignancies. Certain cancer cells grow rapidly in blood plasma, but their growth stopped when vitamin E was added. Administration of vitamin E decreased cancers induced in mice. Cancers produced by giving estrogen, which increases the vitamin E requirement, were also fewer when this vitamin was generously given. The number of breast cancers in mice, has been markedly reduced by vitamin E.

Vitamin C and E can help the body inhibit the activity of the enzyme hyaluronidase, found in cancerous tissue. Vitamin E also increases the oxygenation of cells, which is of great importance both in prevention and treatment of cancer. The use of this vitamin has been found especially valuable in preventing prostate cancer. Latest research studies indicate that the risk of prostate cancer is one third lower in men who take daily supplements of vitamin E than those who do not. In a new study conducted by Dr. Olli P Heinonen of the University of Helsinki in Helsinki, Finland, it was found that of 29,133 Finnish men, those who took 50 milligrams of vitamin E daily, had a 32 per cent lower rate of symptomatic prostate cancer, as compared to those who did not. And the men taking the supplement were 41 per cent less likely to die from the cancer. According to Dr. Heinonen, vitamin E may also enhance the disease-fighting abilities of the immune system.

The study looked at one of the eight naturally occurring forms of vitamin E — alpha-tocopherol — and its most common source in food. The daily recommended intake of eight to ten milligrams can be met by eating a diet abundant in vegetable oils, wheat germ, whole grain cereals and green, leafy vegetables. For the new study, which appeared in an issue of the Journal of the National Cancer Institute, 29,133 male smokers between ages 50 to 69 in Southwestern Finland were randomly chosen and given one of four treatments for five to eight years: vitamin E (50 milligrams daily); beta carotene (20 milligrams daily); vitamin E plus beta carotene; or placebo.

While men who received vitamin E alone, or in combination with beta-carotene, were protected against prostate cancer, beta-carotene alone, did not prevent the disease. In fact, there was a trend towards higher rates of prostate cancer in drinkers who took beta-carotene, the researchers found. Moreover, the reduction in risk associated with vitamin E was seen only among men with more aggressive cancers that resulted in symptoms and not among those with latent, nonsymptomatic prostate cancer. Vitamin E can be administered up to 1,000 I.U. a day.

Plants are nature's remedies and have been used for food and medicine since ancient times. There are herbs for all human afflictions. Herbal traditions have been passed down and refined with scientific understanding. Herbs are valuable sources of natural medicine, vitamins and minerals which have curative effects, when used in the proper way. They act on the blood, metabolism, and all cellular processes. Thus, they are capable of bringing the body into harmony and health.

There are many herbs which have been used for centuries to treat cancer specifically, and as a remedy for the side effects of current cancer treatment, to make them more tolerable. They help in building red and white blood cells, reducing fatigue, eliminating nausea, increasing energy and stimulating the body's immune system to heal itself. Herein are discussed certain herbs which can be beneficially used as a supportive treatment to achieve this.

Alfalfa *(Medico Satina)*

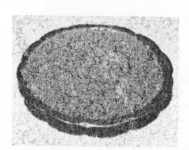

Alfalfa is one the most nutritionally versatile herbs discovered so far. The Arabs who discovered it, called it the "King of kings" of plants and the "Father of all foods". The Persians knew it as one of the nature's most healing grasses. This herb is a valuable source of vitamins A, B, D, E and G. It also has some vitamin C and K. Of special value in alfalfa, is the rich quality, quantity and proper balance of various minerals, which are very much needed for the proper functioning of the different organs of the body.

Alfalfa is an outstanding alkaline food, which makes it a valuable remedy for cancer as it detoxifies the body. These seeds, known as king of sprouts, are very valuable in building up the immune system, for healing cancer, especially stomach cancer and other diseases.

Brahmi *(Herpestis monniera or Bacopa monniera)*

Brahmi, a well known Indian herb can be used as a valuable aid in cancer treatment. This herb increases vitality, strengthens mental faculties and various organs of the body. It thus helps to fight diseases, including cancer. It has been mentioned in the ancient Indian Medical treatise *Charak Samhita*, that this herb cures all kinds of diseases.

Colchicum *(Colchicum luteum)*

The herb Colchicum *(Hirantutiya)*, is a medicine of great repute in Afghanistan and northern India. The medicinal properties of this herb were well known even to the Arabs. The chief constituent of this herb is colchicine, an alkaloid which occurs in the form of yellow flakes, crystals or as whitish yellow amorphous powder. The effect of this alkaloid has been tested on cancerous tissues and it has been found that the drug arrests division of cells of the cancerous tissues and also makes them more susceptible to x-ray treatments. Further experiments are however, being conducted in various laboratories to find out its efficacy in the treatment of cancers.

Ginseng

Ginseng is a wonder herb with outstanding medicinal properties. It has been used in China, Korea, Japan, India and southeast Asia for its vitalizing and restorative power.

Ginseng can be used beneficially in treating cancer as a supportive treatment and in overcoming the after effects of medical treatments. Modern scientific studies on this herb found that it emits a mitogenetic ray, which is considered as an all-natural ultraviolet radiation. Nature has put within ginseng, a process of cellular proliferation via this mitogenetic emission. It is said that this all-natural cellular rejuvenation process stimulates the body's own sluggish process and thereby promotes the youth-building benefit of cellular renewals, which is the key to healing and regenerations.

Holy Basil *(Ocimum sanctum)*

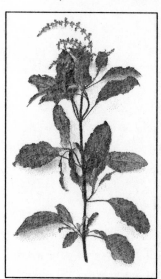

Holy basil, the sacred plant of India, known from the Vedic period, has many medicinal virtues. It is highly beneficial in over-coming stress arising from cancer and the after effects of medical treatment. The basil leaves are regarded as adaptogens or anti-stress agents. Recent studies have shown that the leaves protect against stress significantly. It has been suggested that even healthy persons should chew 12 leaves of basil twice a day, morning and evening, for preventing stress.

Indian Gooseberry *(Emblica officinalis)*

As emphasised in the preceding chapter on vitamins, Vitamin C can greatly help in preventing and controlling cancer. Indian goosebery, which is one of the richest-known sources of vitamin C, can thus be beneficially used in the fight against cancer. Repeated laboratory tests at Coonoor shows that every 100 grams of fresh fruit proves 470 to 680 mgs. of vitamin C.

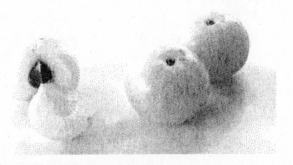

The dehydrated berry will be specially beneficial in controlling cancer. As vitamin C, the value of *amla* increases greatly when the juice is extracted from the fruit. The dehydrated berry provides 2428 to 3470mgs of vitamin C per 100 gms. Even when it is dried in a shade and turned into powder, it retains as much as 1780 to 2660mgs of vitamin C.

Leaves of papaya *(Carica papaya)*

Success in the treatment of cancer has been claimed by a 74-year-old lady from Australia, with the use of the leaves of papaya, a delicious tropical fruit in a letter to "Weekend Bulletin," Gold Coast, Australia. She had undergone surgical operation for her bladder cancer, but the cancer could not be completely removed. While undergoing further treatment in

Brisbane, she used papaya leaves and subsequently used the boiled skin of papaya, when her stock of leaves ran out. After three months when she went to her doctor for a checkup, it was found that her cancer had been healed.

In the U.S.A. too, American scientist Dr Jerry McLaughlin of the University of Purdue, has credited papaya for its cancer fighting role. According to him, he has found a chemical component in the papaya tree that is "one million times stronger than the strongest anti-cancer medicine". There are many reports that cancer sufferers have been healed by drinking papaya leaf concentrate.

Margosa *(Azadirachta indica)*

The use of leaves of margosa, are considered beneficial in the supportive treatment of cancer according to Ayurveda. From the point of view of this system of medicine cancer makes the blood toxic and increases body heat. Margosa leaves help in purifying the blood and in reducing body heat. The patient should therefore, chew ten to twelve margosa leaves daily in the morning.

NATURAL METHODS FOR CONTROLLING CANCER

9

In addition to the dietary treatment prescribed in chapter 4, there are certain natural methods, which can help to control cancer and its symptoms, boost the immune system to promote healing and help overcome the after effects of medical treatment. 'While prescribing treatment through natural methods, the form and sight of the cancer, have no consequence'. The chances of effective treatment and recovery are not influenced by these considerations. The treatment however, is influenced by the amount of morbid matter in the system, which is the root cause of the disease.

The various natural methods found beneficial in the treatment of cancer are discussed herein:

Enema

An enema involves the injection of fluid into the rectum. An enema-can is required for this purpose. This can should be filled with water at 98° F temperature and placed on a suitable hook at a height of four to six feet from the ground. The patient is made to lie on his right side extending his right leg and folding the left leg at right angle. The enema nozzle, lubricated with oil or vaseline, is inserted in the rectum. The water is now allowed to enter into the rectum. Generally, one to two litres of water is injected. The patient may either lie down on his back or walk a little while retaining the water.

After five to 10 minutes, the water can be ejected along with the accumulated morbid matter.

A warm-water enema helps to clean the rectum of accumulated faecal matter and thereby removes toxins from the system. This is not only the safest system for cleaning the bowels, but it also improves the peristalic movement of the bowels thereby relieving constipation.

Enemas are of utmost importance for cancer patients to detoxify the body. As the task of the detoxication is very necessary, especially in the beginning of the treatment, it would be advisable to administer frequent enemas, day and night. Enemas also help against spasms, precordial pain and difficulties resulting from the sudden withdrawl of all intoxicating sedation. Frequent enemas are absolutely necessary in more advanced cases, which are severely intoxicated, and which are intoxicated more with the absorption of the tumour masses and glands.

Dry Friction

Dry friction is an excellent method of keeping the skin in order. This bath can be taken with a rough dry towel or with a moderately soft bristle brush. If a brush is used, the procedure is as follows: take the brush in one hand and begin with the face, neck and chest. Then brush one arm, beginning at the wrist and brushing towards the shoulders. Now brush one foot, then the ankle and leg. Then do the other foot and leg, and next, the hips and central portion of the body. Continue brushing each part until the skin is pink. Use the brush quickly back and forward on every part of the body. If a towel is used, it should be fairly rough, and the same process should be followed as for the use of brush.

Dry friction baths are a very superior means of exciting to increased activity, all the functional processes lying at or near, the surface of the body. Proper activity of the pores of the skin is essential to eradicate morbid methods and waste products from the body through perspiration. Taking this bath regularly will thus enable a person to enjoy a high degree of health, which is very essential for the prevention and treatment of cancer.

Hot Fomentation

This treatment is highly beneficial in case of localised pain during cancer. Hot fomentation is a local application of moist heat by means of clothes wrung from hot water. Select a piece of blanket or flannel large enough to fit over the chest or back. Fold it into a pack, dip it in very hot water, and wring it out as dry as possible. Wrap this in a dry Turkish towel, or any other material thick enough to protect the skin, and apply the whole pack to the area to be treated. Leave the hot pack in place for ten or fifteen minutes or until it is cool. Then rub the area with a small piece of ice or a cold cloth and dry the skin with a rough Turkish towel. The fomentation may be reapplied several times, as desired. Follow this with some massage or heavy rubbing.

Cold Friction Hip-bath

The hip bath is one of the most useful forms of hydrotherapy. As the name suggests, this mode of treatment involves only the hips and the abdominal region below the navel. A special type of tub is used for the purpose. The tub is filled with water in a way that it covers the hips and reaches upto the navel when the patient sits in it. Generally, four to six gallons of water is required. If the special tub is not available, a common tub may be used. A support may be placed under one edge to elevate it by two to three inches.

The water temperature should be 10°C to 18°C. The duration of the bath is usually 10 minutes. The weak patients should, however, take this bath for a duration of five minutes

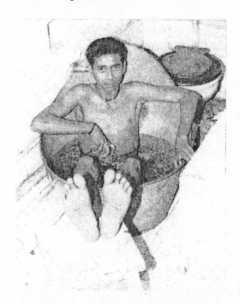

or so. If the patient feels cold, a hot foot immersion should be given with the cold hip bath. The legs should be so adjusted that there is no pressure upon the muscles, ligaments and blood vessels of the knee region.

The patient should rub the abdomen briskly from the navel downwards and across the body with a moderately coarse wet cloth. The legs, feet and upper part of the body should remain completely dry during and after the bath. The patient should undertake moderate exercise after the cold hip bath to warm the body. A cold hip bath is very useful in all diseases, including cancer. It relieves constipation, indigestion and obesity and helps the eliminative organs to function properly. It thus relieves many symptoms of cancer and boosts the immune system for healing.

Cold Friction Sitz-bath

This bath is especially useful in diseases of women, including cancer. The procedure for taking this bath is as follows: fill an ordinary bath-tub with cold water to a depth of four inches or so, and sit in it so that the feet, the seat, and the sexual organs are for the most part in the water. Only the seat and feet should touch the bottom of the tub, while the knees are always above the water.

The knees are now spread apart and the water is vigorously dashed over the abdomen with the hollow of the hand. The throwing of the water is followed by a brisk rubbing of the abdomen with both hands. After this process has been carried on for a while, all the parts immersed in the water, except the sexual organs which, should be rubbed vigorously with the open hand. Then get out and dry with a rough towel. The rubbing dry is a good exercise and improves the condition of the skin.

It is especially recommended for heightening the strength of the organs lying in the region of the hips. It greatly increases the circulation in these parts, hardens and strengthens the tissues, and is an important adjunct to the building of nervous vigour and sexual strength. It has a decidedly invigorating effect upon the whole sexual organism, and it greatly assists in influencing the regular movement of the bowels. This bath should not be taken during menstural periods. Friction sitz bath is a very superior method to keep the body healthy, increase energy and vitality and to boost the immune system, which are very necessary in preventing and controlling cancer.

Steam Bath

Steam bath is one of the most important time-tested water treatments, which induces perspiration in a most natural way. The patient, clad in minimum loin cloth or underwear, is made to sit on a stool inside a specially designed cabinet. Before entering the cabinet, the patient should drink one or two glasses of cold water and protect the head with a cold towel. The duration of steam bath is generally 10 to 20 minutes or until profuse perspiration takes place. A cold shower should be taken immediately after the bath.

If the patient feels giddy or uneasy during the steam bath, he or she should immediately be taken out and given a glass of cold water and the face washed with cold water.

The steam bath helps to eliminate morbid matter from the surface of the skin. It also improves circulation of blood and tissue activity. It relieves rheumatism, gout, uric acid problems, jaundice, obesity and many symptoms of cancer. The steam bath is helpful in all forms of chronic toxemias, which is the root cause of cancer.

When there is unbearable pain in cancer, this bath should be taken frequently during the day. The pain is greatly relieved by taking this bath and the patient feels relieved. In two or three days time, the internal gangrenous inflammation begins to travel downward.

Neutral Immersion Bath

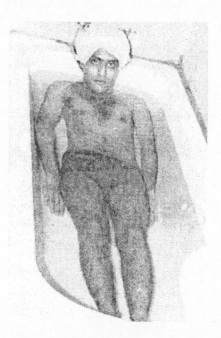

This is also known as full tub bath. It is administered in a bath tub which should be properly fitted with hot and cold water connection. This bath can be given from 15 to 60 minutes at a temperature ranging from 26°C to 28°C. It can be given for long duration, without any ill-effects, as the water temperature is akin to the body temperature. The neutral bath diminishes the pulse rate without modifying respiration. This treatment is the best sedative. It also excites activity of both the skin and the kidneys and helps built up health. This treatment is therefore, very useful in controlling cancer and its symptoms.

Relaxation Method

It is essential for cancer patients to learn how to relax physically and mentally. In relaxation, the muscles work more efficiently. Fatigue is also completely relieved in a very short time as the venous blood circulation is promoted throughout the body. The best method of relaxation is to practice *shavasana* or 'the dead pose.'

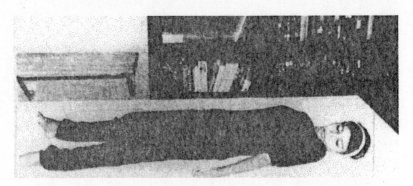

The procedure for practising this asana is as follow: lie flat on your back, feet comfortably apart, arms and hands extended about six inches from the body, palms upwards and fingers half-folded. Close your eyes. Begin by consciously and gradually relaxing every part and each muscle of the body, i.e. feet, legs, calves, knees, thighs, abdomens, hips, back, hands, arms, chest, shoulders, neck, head and face. Relax yourself completely, feeling as if your whole body is lifeless. Now concentrate your mind on breathing rhythmically as slowly and effortlessly as possible. This creates a state of complete relaxation. Remain motionless in this position, relinquishing all responsibilities and worries for 10 to 15 minutes. Discontinue the exercise when your legs grow numb. This asana relaxes the mind and soothens the nervous system. It is thus very beneficial in controlling cancer and its symptoms and to create a feeling of well being.

Meditation

Cancer patients should also meditate frequently and explore and develop their spiritual interests. The state of meditation or *dhyana* is achieved when the mind is trained to concentrate on an outer or inner object, long enough for all distractions to be eliminated, until the stream of thoughts flows in a single direction without interruption. The body is silently resting in this state. The only sign of life is breathing. The hypothalamus recharges its energy during meditation.

Meditation helps eliminate emotional conflict, inner discord and psychological tension. It completely purifies the mind and frees it from unconscious obstructions. The most common traditional method consists in concentrating one's attention on an object of personal value or an universal symbol.

Each person, according to his faith, usually chooses an elevated thought or spiritual symbol upon which he prefers to meditate. It is essential to adopt a comfortable and firm posture. Otherwise meditation will not be possible. To adopt a firm posture means to hold one-self in such a way that one is conscious of the body. The slightest discomfort in such a posture will prove a constant distraction to the mind; one should therefore choose the position that allows one to remain still for a long time without feeling discomfort. The spine and head should be kept very straight, but without being strained. *Padmasana* is considered to be the ideal posture for practising meditation. Meditation constitutes a very effective method to control symptoms of cancer, boost immune system for healing and overcome after effects of medical treatment.

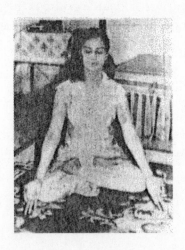

Other helpful natural methods for the treatment of cancer include plenty of rest, complete freedom from worries and mental stress and plenty of fresh pure air day and night. If the patient is strong, he can undertake lots of exercise and walking. He should generally adopt a health-strengthening mode of living.

TYPES OF CANCER
(THEIR SYMPTOMS, CAUSES AND TREATMENTS)

10

There is no organ in the body in which cancer cannot develop. There are thus many types of cancers. The clinical and experimental observations of the past many years have shown that cancer of different tissues, although they possess many common features, behave differently from one another. The difference depends on the site of development, the tissue of origin and the character of the cells, which go to make up the cancer. In this chapter, some more important types of cancer are described, along with their symptom, causes, and treatments, medical as well as natural.

Bladder Cancer

Bladder cancer is a disease in which cancer cells are found in the bladder. The bladder is a hollow organ in the lower part of the abdomen, which stores urine. It is shaped like a small balloon, and it has a muscular wall that allows it to get larger or smaller. Urine is the liquid waste made by the kidneys when they clean the blood. The urine passes from the two kidneys into the bladder through two tubes called urethras. When the bladder is emptied during urination, the urine goes from the bladder to the outside of the body through another tube called the urethra.

Symptoms: The most common symptom of bladder cancer is the blood in urine, known as hematuria in medical parlance. Other symptoms are burning or pain on urination, frequent passage of urine, or an urge to pass urine but no urine is passed. Advance cases of bladder cancer are characterised by loss of weight, tiredness, and abdominal, pelvic, or back pain.

Causes: Certain environmental factors seem to increase the risk of bladder cancer. These factors include cigarette smoking and exposure to naphthalene, benzidine, aniline dyes, and chemicals used in rubber and leather processing.

Diagnosis: Bladder cancer can be detected by laboratory tests of the urine, to ascertain the presence of cancer cells. These tests can also detect occult blood in urine. The doctor may also do an internal examination by inserting gloved fingers into the vagina or rectum to feel for lumps. In case of suspected malignancy, a special x-ray called an intravenous pyelogram (IVP) is used to locate the cancer.

Treatment: Medical treatment of bladder cancer consists of surgery or taking out the cancer in an operation; radiation therapy, which involves using high-dose x-rays or other high-energy rays to kill cancer cells and shrink tumours; and chemotherapy which uses drugs to kill cancer cells. Bladder cancer is curable, if diagnoised early.

Natural Methods: The most important natural treatment for bladder cancer is warm water enema to eradicate toxins from the body, which is the root cause of the disease. Enema should be taken twice daily. In advanced cases, it should be taken more frequently. Certain other natural methods can be implied to relieve pain arising from cancer, strengthen immune system for healing and improve the quality of life. These methods include daily morning dry friction, cold sitz or hip bath, occasional steam bath, massage, yogic asanas, relaxation techniques and meditation. Some nutritionists believe that bladder cancer can be prevented by an appropriate diet. A low intake of vitamin A is generally associated with the increased risk of this type of cancer. It is therefore, advisable to take vitamin A-rich foods such as yellow or orange fruits and vegetables, as well as dark green vegetables. The patient should give up smoking completely, if it is habitual, and minimise exposure to possible cancer causing agents. Protective equipment should be used by those engaged in occupations, which require exposure to harmful chemicals.

Hair dyes have also been suspected as a possible cause for this type of cancer. It is therefore, advisable to use semipermanent, light-coloured dyes as a precautionary measure.

Bone Cancer

Bone Cancer is a relatively rare malignancy. It can occur at any age. More often, it strikes during childhood or adolescence. There are several different types of bone cancer. Cancer occurring in the breast, prostate, thyroid, lung, or kidney often spreads to the bones through the process known as metastasis.

Symptom: The most common symptom of bone cancer is intense pain which cannot be relieved with painkillers. Other symptoms are unexplained fractures, fatigue and loss of appetite and weight. There is also a persistent low-grade fever and swelling, depending on the tumour site.

Causes: Cancers, which arise elsewhere and spread to the bones, as mentioned above, are actually more common than primary bone cancer.

Diagnosis: In most cases, the bone tumour is first discovered by routine X-ray. A special bone scan can be done in cases where a new bone is being formed.

Treatment: Surgery is the usual medical treatment for bone cancer. Occasionally, the tumour can be removed along with a margin of healthy tissue; followed by radiation treatments and chemotherapy, to remove any remaining cancer cells.

Natural Methods: Natural methods can be implied as supportive treatments to the medical treatment being carried out by the specialists. The most important of these methods is warm water enema to eliminate morbid matter from the system. In advanced cases, repeated enemas will be necessary to detoxify the body. Other natural methods include daily dry friction and sitz bath. These methods would help reduce pain and relieve after-effects of medical treatment. Gentle exercise and simple yogic *asanas* can help regenerate healthy bone after radiation treatments. However, the doctor must be consulted before adopting any exercise. The patient should take easily digestible foods, with emphasis on foods high in protein, calcium and the various other nutrients aimed at boosting the immune system for healing.

Brain Cancer

Brain Cancer is a disease in which cancer cells begin to grow in the tissues of the brain. The brain controls memory and learning, senses and emotion. It also controls other parts of the body, including muscles, organs and blood vessels.

Often, cancer found in the brain starts elsewhere in the body and spreads to the brain. This is called brainz metastasis.

Of the primary brain cancers, gliomas are the most prevalent, accounting for about 45 per cent of cases. Gliomas and other primary brain cancers seldom metastasise. Their rate of growth varies greatly. Some may be present for years without causing any problems, while others are fatal.

Symptoms: Symptoms of brain cancer includes severe or persistent headaches, personality changes, increased irritability and moodiness, unusual sleepiness, unexplained nausea and vomiting, paralysis, and balance problems, with difficulty in walking and speaking. There may also be some defects of the senses, including hearing, vision, speech, taste and smell.

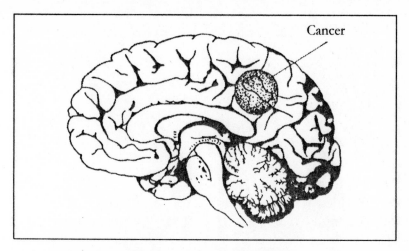

Causes: According to modern medical system, causes of brain tumour are largely unknown. There is, however, some evidence that points to environmental factors as a cause of brain cancer. The increase in incidence of this type of cancer may be linked to a viral infection or possibly exposure, to radiation or certain chemicals.

Diagnosis: The presence of brain cancer is confirmed by various imaging techniques, which usually involve X-rays of the skull and CT scans or MRI. A biopsy of the tumour cells is necessary to ascertain whether the tumour is malignant or not.

Treatment: The medical treatments of brain tumour consist of radiation therapy, surgery, or a combination of both and chemotherapy. In some cases, the entire tumour can be removed to effect complete cure.

Natural Methods: Natural methods can be implied to relieve pain and other symptoms of cancer and to boost the immune system for healing. These methods include warm water enema, dry friction, sitz bath, relaxation methods, especially *shavasana* and meditation. They may be combined with chemotherapy and radiation as part of the overall treatment program.

Breast Cancer

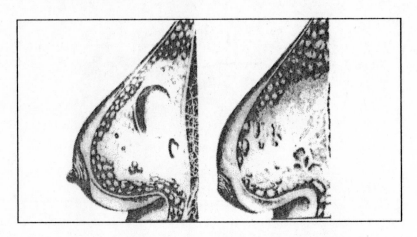

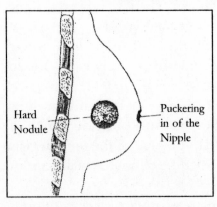

Hard Nodule   Puckering in of the Nipple

Breast Cancer is the most common malignancy in women and the most important cause of death among females due to cancer. It is a disease in which cancer cells are found in the tissues of the breast. Each breast has 15-20 sections called lobes, which have many smaller sections called lobules. The lobes and lobules are connected by thin tubes called ducts. The most common type of breast cancer is ductal cancer. It is found in the cells of the ducts.

Symptoms: Cancer that begins in the lobes or lobules is called lobular cancer. It is more often found in both breasts than other types of breast cancer. Inflammatory breast cancer is an uncommon type of cancer. In this disease, the breast is warm, red, and swollen.

Causes: The risk of breast cancer increases with age,

especially after menopause. The risk is also higher among those women who have their first child after the age of 30 or have never had children, have already have had cancer in one breast, had early menstrual periods or late menopause. Mothers who do not breast feed their babies are also at a greater risk of this cancer.

Some studies suggest a link between a high-fat diet and breast cancer. Hereditary factors also influence the incidence of this disease – it constitutes approximately five to ten per cent of all breast cancer cases. The genes in cells carry the hereditary information that is received from a person's parents. Several genes have been found to be defective in some breast cancer patients. Relatives of breast cancer patients who carry these defective genes may be more likely to develop breast or ovarian cancer.

Hormonal contraceptives may be another factor to consider. Research findings suggest a link between the use of contraceptive and a slightly increased risk of developing breast cancer.

Diagnosis: Early detection of breast cancer is the essential factor for the patients survival as early localised malignancies are curable in most cases. The Canadian Cancer Society recommends that all women at the age of 40 and above should undertake self-examination of their breasts. In such self-examination, many women find benign lumps and most of them are also able to detect breast cancer. Breast examination by a physician is recommended every three years between the ages of 20 and 40 and annually, thereafter. However, the most important methods of early detection of breast cancer in women above 50 is mammography which can locate suspicious areas of calcification, which is the common sign of cancer. If any suspicious areas are found by mammography or physical examination, a biopsy is necessary to rule out cancer.

Treatment: The chance of recovery and choice of treatment depend on the stage of the cancer – whether it is just in the breast or has spread to other places in the body, the type of breast cancer, certain characteristics of the cancer cells, and whether the cancer is found in the other breast. A woman's age, weight, menopausal status and general health can also affect the choice of treatment.

Medically, four types of treatments are used. These are surgery, radiation therapy, chemotherapy and hormone therapy. Hormone therapy involves using drugs that change the way hormones work or taking out organs that make hormones, such as the ovaries.

In most cases of breast cancer, surgery is employed to remove the cancer from the breast. Usually, some of the lymph nodes under the arm are also taken out for biopsy.

Natural Methods: Certain natural methods can be used to relieve symptoms of breast cancer and the after effects of medical treatment. These include warm water enema, daily dry friction, sitz bath, relaxation methods, especially *shavasana* and meditation. These methods will help boost the functioning of the immune system and improve the quality of life. Some nutritionists recommend the use of daily supplements of beta carotene (precursor to vitamin A), vitamins C and E, for preventing breast cancer, as well as for retarding its progress. However, studies suggest that foods high in these antioxidants are more effective. Good sources of beta carotene are orange and dark green vegetables and yellow and orange fruits. Vitamin C is contained in many fruits and vegetables, especially citrus fruits. Rich vegetarian sources of vitamin E are wheat germ, legumes and vegetable oils. Some studies suggest that a low-fat diet may cut the risk of breast cancer and its recurrence. Such a regimen requires limiting the intake of all fats, especially those from animals, as well as animal protein, while increasing foods high in fibre, such as whole-grain products and fresh fruits and vegetables.

Colon and Rectal Cancer

Cancer of the colon, a common form of cancer, is a disease in which cancer cells are found in the tissues of the colon. The colon is part of the body's digestive system. The purpose of the digestive system is to remove nutrients like vitamins, minerals, carbohydrates, fats, proteins and water from the foods eaten and to store the waste until it passes out of the body. The digestive system is made up of the esophagus, stomach and the small and large intestines. The last six feet of the intestine is called the large bowel or colon.

Symptoms: The main symptoms of colon and rectal cancer are a change in bowel habits and bleeding from the rectum.

Causes: It is known that a single gene is responsible for about one in every seven colon cancers. Other risk factors include the presence of colon polyps, inflammatory bowel disease and certain other kinds of cancer, especially of the breast, uterus and ovaries.

Screening tests (such as a rectal examination, proctoscopy, and colonoscopy) are the methods implied to ascertain presents or otherwise of colon and rectal cancer.

The patients who are at age 50, who have a family history of cancer of the colon, rectum or of the female organs, who have had small non cancerous growths in the colon, or who have a history of ulcerative colitis are more prone to colon and rectal cancer.

Diagnosis: The diagnosis usually begin with rectal examination. In this examination, the doctor, wearing thin gloves, puts a greased finger into the rectum and gently feels for lumps. The doctor may then check the material collected from the rectum to see if there is any blood in it.

The doctor may also want to look inside the rectum and lower colon with a special instrument called a sigmoidoscope or a proctosigmoidoscope to know more about the colon and rectal cancers. Some pressure may be felt, but usually with no pain.

If any abnormal tissue is found, the doctor will need to cut out a small piece and look at it under the microscope to see if there are any cancer cells (biopsy).

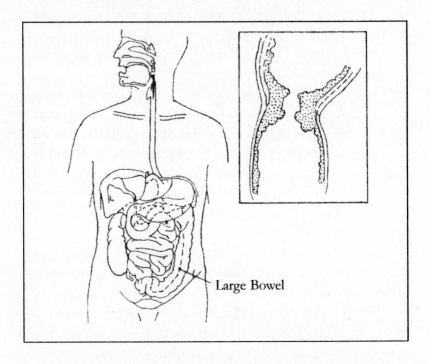

Large Bowel

Treatment: The chance of recovery and choice of treatment depend on the stage of the cancer – whether it is just in the inner lining of the colon or if it has spread to other places, and the patient's general state of health.

Medically three kinds of treatments for colon cancer are available. These are surgery, radiation therapy and chemotherapy.

Natural Methods: Natural methods can play a supportive role to medical treatment. The pain and other symptoms of cancers, as well as the after effects of treatment can be controlled through warm water enema, cold sitz or hip bath, hot fomentation, daily dry friction, relaxation technique and meditation.

The risk of colon and rectal cancer can be considerably reduced by adhering to a diet that is low in animal fat and high in fibre. Dietary fibre can help prevent constipation by producing soft, bulky stool, which can pass easily and quickly through the colon. This will protect greatly against colon cancer, according to some recent research studies. More fibre to diet should, however, be introduced gradually, as sudden increase may result in digestive disorders. Recent research studies have also shown that liberal intake of Vitamin A, C and E, as well as calcium, may lower the risk of developing colon cancer.

Other helpful measure in preventing colon and rectal cancer are eating a low-fat diet, eating more fibre-rich foods, a liberal intake of green vegetables and fresh fruit daily, controlling the caloric intake at the level necessary to maintain ideal weight and ensuring a well-balanced diet based mainly on alkaline-foods.

Esophageal Cancer

Cancer of the esophagus is a disease in which cancer cells are found in the tissues of the esophagus. The esophagus is the hollow tube that carries food and liquid from the throat to the stomach.

Symptoms: The most common symptom of cancer of the esophagus is difficulty in swallowing. Pain may be felt while swallowing and also from behind the breastbone.

Causes: The most important causes of esophageal cancer are high intake of spicy foods, animal fats and smoking. Vitamin deficiency may also cause injury of esophageal lining and ultimately lead to cancer.

Diagnosis: Barium meal x-ray is the most common way to diagnose this cancer. A patient is made to drink a liquid containing barium, which makes the esophagus easier to see in the x-ray.

A doctor may also loom at the inside of the esophagus with a thin, lighted tube called esophagoscope. This test is called an esophagoscopy. If the tissue is abnormal, biospy will be necessary.

Treatment: The chance of recovery and choice of treatment depend on the stage of the cancer and the patient's general state of health. Medical treatments for esophageal cancer are surgery, radiation therapy and chemotherapy. However, surgery is the most common treatment for this cancer.

Natural Methods: Some Natural methods can be implied for managing pain and mitigating the symptoms and side effects of medical treatment. These include warm water enema, daily dry friction, cold sitz or hip bath, relaxation methods and meditation.

Ginger may be used to prevent or minimise nausea, a common complication of radiation treatment and chemotherapy.

Gall Bladder Cancer

Cancer of the gall bladder is an uncommon cancer. It is a disease in which cancer cells are found in the tissues of the gall bladder. The gall bladder is a pear-shaped organ that lies just under the liver in the upper abdomen. Bile, a fluid made by the liver, is stored in the gall bladder. When food is digested in the stomach and the intestines, bile is released from the gall bladder through a tube called the bile duct that connects the gall bladder and liver to the first part of the small intestine. The bile helps to digest fat.

Gall bladder cancer mainly affects people in their late

sixties and seventies and is somewhat more common among woman than men. Between 70 and 80 per cent of those who have the cancer also have chronic gallstones and cholecystitis or gall bladder inflammation.

Symptoms: The symptoms of gall bladder cancer are pain above the stomach, unexplained loss of weight, and jaundice.

Causes: The chief cause of gall bladder cancer is gallstones. Prolonged irritation caused by gallstones rubbing against the gall bladder can lead to this cancer.

Diagnosis: An ultrasound examination, CT scan and MRI are the usual tests done to detect gall bladder cancer. However, normally the cancer cannot be found unless the patient has surgery. During surgery, a cut is made in the abdomen so that the gall bladder and other nearby organs and tissues can be examined.

Treatment: The chance of recovery and choice of treatment depend on the stage of cancer and on the patient's general health. Medical treatments implied for gall bladder cancer are surgery, Radiation therapy, and chemotherapy. Surgery, however, is the most common treatment for this cancer.

Natural Methods: Pain, stress and other symptom resulting from gall bladder cancer can be relieved by warm water enema, hot fomentation, dry friction, hip bath, relaxation techniques and meditation. Loss of appetite being common in this cancer, the patient should take frequent small meals based on alkaline-forming light foods like fruit and vegetables and their juices, at the start of the treatment. Special enriched supplements may also be taken to prevent excessive weight loss as fats would be difficult to digest.

As the presence of gallstones is usually associated with gall bladder cancer, measures can be taken to prevent the formation of gallstones. In case of elevated cholesterol levels, a cholesterol-lowering diet may be adopted. Such a diet should be high in starches and fibre. Fat intake may be restricted to 20 per cent or less of total calorie intake. If the person is overweight, he should follow a sensible low calorie diet and undertake physical exercises to lose weight gradually. Smoking, if habitual, should be given up completely, as cigarette smoking has been associated with gallstone attack. Women who have had the stones should avoid birth control pills and estrogen replacement, because high levels of this hormone have been associated with gall bladder disease.

Kidney Cancer

Renal cell cancer, also called cancer of the kidney or renal adenocarcinoma, is a disease in which cancer cells are found in certain tissues of the kidney. It is one of the less common kinds of cancer. It occurs more often in men than in women.

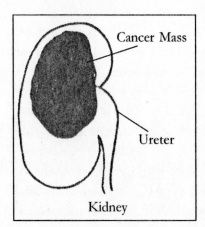

Kidney cancer most often originates in the nephrons, the filtering units of the kidney, and account for 85 per cent of cases. This cancer can strike at any age, but it is most common between ages 40 and 60. Cancer of the renal pelvis, which starts in the central part of the kidney, frequently spreads to the urethras, the tubes that carry urine from the kidneys, and to the bladder.

Symptoms: The symptoms of kidney cancer are blood in the urine, a lump in the abdomen and pain in the side that doesn't go away. Other symptoms are tiredness, loss of appetite, unexplained loss of weight and anemia.

Causes: The main cause of kidney cancer is unknown, although heredity is thought to play a role. Cigarette smoking and exposure to asbestos increase the risk of renal cell carcinoma. Persons on long-terms kidney dialysis also have increased incidence of kidney cancer.

Diagnosis: The doctor will usually feel the abdomen for lumps and order a special x-ray called an intravenous pyelogram (IVP) which enables him to see the kidney more clearly on the x-ray. Other methods for diagnosis are ultrasound. CT scan and MRI.

Treatment: There are five types of treatment for renal cell cancer. The chance of recovery and choice of treatment depend on the stage of the cancer and the patient's general state of health.

Medical treatments include surgery, chemotherapy, radiation therapy, hormone therapy and biological therapy. The last-named treatment uses the body's immune system to fight cancer.

Natural Methods: Warm water enema is one of the most important natural methods to eradicate morbid matter from the system, which is the chief cause of cancer. Other natural methods can be implied as supportive treatment to relieve the symptoms of cancer and the after-effects of medical treatment, as well as to boost the immune system. These methods include daily dry friction, hot fomentation, friction, sitz or hip bath, relaxation methods, especially *shavasana* and meditation. These techniques may be especially beneficial as renal cell cancer responds to anything that bolsters the immune system. Some leaves of holi basil can also be chewed to reduce stress.

Although diet has no impact on kidney cancer itself, dietary changes may reduce the risk of contracting it among people who have chronic kidney stones.

Kidney cancer can be prevented through dietary changes

as indicated in chapter 4 on diet, as well as by avoiding smoking and by wearing a protective mask if working with naphthalene, aniline dyes and other potentially harmful chemicals. Anyone with congenital kidneys or urinary tract abnormalities should undergo frequent screening examinations to detect possible kidney cancer in the early stages when it is possible to treat it successfully.

Leukaemia

Leukaemia is a term used to describe several types of blood cancer. It comes from the Greek word meaning white blood. The name refers to whitish or pale-pink blood, as leukaemia patients have high numbers of abnormal white cells. Although leukaemia affects all types of blood cells, bone marrow and other blood-producing structures, the white cells, or lymphocytes, are most affected.

Commonly known as blood cancer, leukaemia is a serious disorder of the blood-forming tissues. There are a number of different varieties of leukaemia. Fortunately, none of these are common compared with other diseases.

Symptoms: The main symptoms of leukaemia are weakness, fatigue, lack of appetite and weight loss. There may be anaemia or loss of red blood cells due to the bone marrow being overcrowded with white blood cells. The spleen is usually large and tender. There may be pain in the bones and haemorrhages in the skin in various parts of the body. The white blood count may rise from the normal 7,000 to 25,000 or even 50,000. In some cases, it may rise to over 200,000. The outcome depends largely on the type of leukaemia.

Causes: The cause of this disease is still unknown. It may be due to some virus. This has been experimented with mice, but not yet in man. It may follow excessive exposure to X-rays and certain chemicals, particularly those related to the benzene group.

Diagnosis: Microscopic examination of blood will reveal abnormal cells, raising the suspicion of leukaemia. This can be confirmed by a bone marrow biopsy. The specific type of leukaemia can also be ascertained in this matter.

Treatment: Medically, leukaemias are usually treated with intensive chemotherapy, using various combinations of anticancer drugs. Radiation therapy is also used frequently. Other treatments include transfusions of red cells, platelets and occasionally, white blood cells. Specialists are also recommending bone marrow transplants for a growing number of patients.

Natural Methods: Certain natural methods can be implied as a supportive treatment to relieve symptoms of cancer, enhance the feeling to well-being and promote healing by strengthening the immune system. These methods may include repeated warm water enema, dry friction bath and cold hip bath everyday, relaxation techniques and meditation.

Liver Cancer

Cancer that originates in the liver is uncommon worldwide. However, it is one of the most common malignancies. Most of liver cancers come from elsewhere.

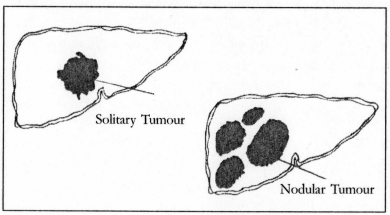

Solitary Tumour

Nodular Tumour

Hence, the earlier the diagnosis is made, the better the patient's chance of recovery. Once the cancer has begun to grow within the liver, it spreads rapidly, eventually causing jaundice and swelling in the distant tissues. The condition resembles cirrhosis, but is far more serious.

Symptoms: In its early stages, liver cancer usually has no noticeable symptoms. When symptoms develop, they initially include fatigue, loss of appetite and weight loss and vague discomfort in the upper-right abdomen, possibly with a spread of pain to the shoulder and back. As the cancer progresses, jaundice, which is marked by yellowing of the skin, whites of eyes and mucous membranes, develops. In its advanced stages, liver cancer produces ascetics, noticeable swelling caused by fluid retention in the abdomen. When it begins in the stomach or large bowel, the liver may soon be involved, mainly because the blood flows toward the liver all the digestive organs including the pancreas and gall bladder. This is referred to as metastatic carcinoma. In other words, the cancer has come from some other part of the body.

Causes: The precise cause of liver cancer is not known. However, chronic hepatitis is considered to be major precipitating factor, as is cirrhosis, a disease in which scar tissue replaces normal liver cells. Other factors which may contribute to liver cancer are occupational exposure to vinyl chloride and similarly toxic chemicals, the use of synthetic testosterone and other anabolic steroids to build muscle mass and alcoholism. Some experts believe that environmental and cultural factors play a strong role in its development.

Diagnosis: Palpating, or pressing, on the upper abdomen may reveal that the liver is enlarged and hard, forming a lump below the rib cage on the right side. Other methods which can be employed to diagnose the disease are X-rays, CT scans, MRI, and ultrasound studies. However, a biopsy is necessary for correct diagnosis.

Treatment: A local tumour, such as hepatocellular carcinoma, the most common type of liver cancer, can be removed by surgery, which may sometimes result in a cure. Chemotherapy may be employed after surgery. In case of inoperative and advanced cases, radiation therapy may relieve pain and prolong life.

Natural Methods: A low-salt diet can help to reduce fluid accumulation. May nutritionists advocate supplements of beta carotene, a precursor of vitamin A that is believed to suppress cancer cells, but studies indicate that food sources are more effective than pills. These include deep green or orange vegetables, such as broccoli, spinach, sweet potato, and carrots. Some experts also recommend tomatoes, watermelon, and red peppers, as they contain lycopene, which seems to have some anticancer potential.

Other natural methods can be employed to relieve pains create a sense of well-being and boost immune system for healing. These methods include dry friction bath, cold hip bath, yogic asanas, relaxation techniques especially *shavasana*, and meditation.

Lung Cancer

Cancer of the lung has become very widespread today. In fact, it is increasing more rapidly than any other type of cancer. Primary cancer of the lung, also known as, bronchogenic carcinoma, begins within the lung or one of the bronchial tubs. More men die from cancer of the lung today than any other form of cancer. Unfortunately, by the time the patient is aware of his true condition, the disease may have already reached advance stage. This is what makes cancer of the lung quite dangerous.

Symptoms: The earliest and most important symptoms of lung cancer is a chronic cough. Even the so-called "cigarette cough" may be a danger signal. Any cough lasting more than three weeks should be thoroughly investigated. Another symptom is wheezing. The patient may notice this first when he is lying quietly in bed just before dropping off to sleep. Later there may be chest pains, followed by night sweats as the tumour mass cuts off the normal drainage from the lungs. Other symptoms of lung cancer are loss of weight, fine streaks of blood being coughed up from the bronchial tubes. Some cases of so-called "virus pneumonia" have later been shown to be due to cancer of the lung.

Causes: Heavy smoking is the most important cause of lung cancer. At the present rate, one heavy cigarette smoker out of every ten will die of lung cancer. Even those who smoke only a few cigarettes a day run some risk of developing this disease, but in men who smoke two packets a day, the risk is extremely high. Some substance, perhaps the tar that is always present in tobacco leaves, seems to irritate the lining of the bronchial tubes. This substance has long been known to produce cancer when applied to the backs of mice and other experimental animals. Contaminated atmosphere also plays some role in development of lung cancer.

Diagnosis: There is no effective screening test to detect

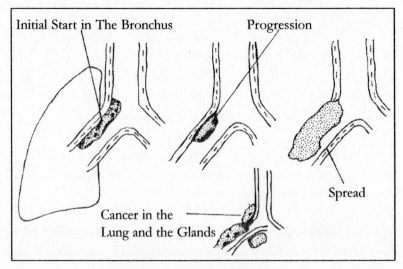

Initial Start in The Bronchus   Progression

Cancer in the
Lung and the Glands   Spread

lung cancer. Sometimes laboratory tests of sputum may detect abnormal cells in the early stages of the disease, but it may be extremely difficult to pin point the exact location. Generally, by the time lung cancer can be detected by chest x-rays, it would have spread to other parts of the body. If symptoms indicate possibility of lung cancer, the diagnostic methods may include thorough physical examination, laboratory tests, chest x-ray, CT scan and bronchoscopy. The last-named test enables direct examination of the lung. A sample of tissue can also be extracted by this method for biopsy.

Treatment: Once the diagnosis of lung cancer is made, surgery is perhaps the only effective method of treatment. The chest is opened very wide so that the surgeon can examine all areas. If cancer is found in only one lobe lung, it may be possible to remove this portion completely. Other medical treatments include radiation to shrink tumour and chemotherapy in case of spread of the disease beyond lymph nodes. In many cases, a combination of different treatments may be useful.

Natural Methods: Warm water enema should be taken as frequently as possible to remove toxins from the body. Other natural methods can be implied as a supportive treatment to relieve pain, and other symptoms of cancer, to overcome after effects of medical treatments and to boost immune system for healing. These methods include hot fomentation, daily dry friction bath, friction sitz or hip bath, relaxation methods and meditation.

Many nutritionists believe that daily supplements of antioxidant vitamins, beta carotene and vitamins C and E can help prevent lung cancer. Studies, however, indicate that food sources of these vitamins are more protective than vitamin supplements. Foods rich in these vitamins are yellow and orange fruits and orange and dark green vegetables especially cruciferous, such as cabbage, cauliflower and Brussel sprouts.

The best approach to avoid lung cancer is to adopt measures to prevent it. Smoking, if habitual, must be given up completely. Research studies show that within weeks of quitting smoking, suspicious precancerous lesions begin to heal and in five to ten years, the risk of cancer in ex-smokers is only slightly higher than that of non-smokers. Even in those who have lung cancer, giving up smoking and living in a smoke-free environment, may slow down the growth of the cancer.

Lymphoma

Lymphomas are malignant tumours of the lymph system, which is a part of the immune system. It is made up of thin tubes that branch, like blood vessels, into all parts of the body, including the skin. Lymph vessels carry lymph, a colourless, watery fluid that contains lymphocytes, the infection-fighting substances.

There are several types of lymphoma. The most common types are called Hodgkin's disease and non-Hodgkin's lymphoma. These types of lymphoma usually start in the lymph nodes and the spleen.

Symptoms: The most common general symptom of lymphoma is a painless enlargement of one or more lymph nodes in the neck, groin and armpit. In case of Hodgkin's disease, there is low-grade fever and night sweats. Some patients of non-Hodgkin lymphoma also develop skin rashes, enlarged tonsils and abdominal swelling.

Causes: According to modern medical system, the cause of many lymphomas is unknown. Some lymphomas are linked to viruses. In recent years, the HIV (AIDs) virus has been linked to a type of non-Hodgkin's lymphoma.

Diagnosis: In case of suspicion, the doctor will palpate or feel, all lymph nodes that lie close to the surface of the body. Any suspicious growth will be removed for biopsy. Other diagnostic techniques like laparotomy and lymphangiography may be adopted in case of Hodgkin's disease. Bone marrow studies and CT scan may be necessary in case of non-Hodgkin's lymphoma.

Treatment: The chance of recovery and choice of treatment depend on the stage of the cancer as to whether it is just in the skin or has spread to other places in the body and the patient's general state of health. Radiation therapy is the usual method of treatment for Hodgkin's disease. A combination of radiation therapy and chemotherapy and possibly surgery, may be necessary in some cases. Radiation therapy is also often implied for non-Hodgkin's lymphomas. Chemotherapy may be necessary where the disease has spread.

Natural Method: Certain natural methods may be implied as a supportive therapy to relieve pain and other symptoms of lymphomas, to boost immune system for healing and to overcome the after-effects of medical treatment. These methods may include frequent warm-water enemas, daily dry friction, cold hip bath and neutral immersion bath. Relaxation techniques and meditation are also very beneficial.

Melanoma

Melanoma is a disease of the skin in which cancer cells are found in the cells that colour the skin (melanocytes). Melanoma usually occurs in adults, but it may occasionally be found in children and adolescents. The skin protects the body against heat, light, infection and injury. It is made up of two main layers known as epidermis, the top layer and dermis, the inner layer. Melanocytes are found in the epidermis and they contain melanin, which gives the skin its colour.

Melanoma is the most fatal type of skin cancer. Unlike other types of skin cancer, it frequently spreads through other parts of the body like lungs, brain, liver, and other internal organs.

Symptoms: The common symptoms of melanoma are change in the size, shape, or colour of a mole, oozing or bleeding from a mole, or a mole that feels itchy, hard, lumpy, swollen, or tender to the touch. Melanoma can also appear on the body as a new mole. Men most often get this disease on the trunk or on the head or neck, while women most often get it on the arms and legs.

Causes: The most common cause of melanoma is excessive exposure to sun. This is especially true in case of people with light-skin, as their skin is more susceptible to sun burn. Other causes of this cancer are occupational exposure to coal tar, pitch, creosote, arsenic compounds and radium. Heredity also plays a role in causing this cancer.

Diagnosis: Melanoma can be diagnoised by careful examination of the skin to see whether a mole or pigmented area looks normal or not. If it is abnormal, biopsy will be necessary.

Treatment: Medically, four kinds of treatments are available for melanoma. These are surgery, chemotherapy, radiation therapy and biological therapy.

Natural Methods: Natural methods can be successfully implied to control pain and stress arising from medical treatment and to strengthen the body's immune system for healing. These methods include frequent warm water enemas, daily dry friction, hip or sitz bath, deep breathing exercises, relaxation techniques and meditation.

It would be advisable to minimise the intake of omega-6 fatty acids like corn oil, safflower oil and sunflower oil and take more of the omega-3 type fat. When the cells have too much omega-6 fat and not enough omega-3, the production of prostaglandins goes into overdrive. This encourages the onset and growth of skin tumours.

An international conference on melanoma in 1989, concluded that eating butter, with a higher ratio of omega-3 to omega-6, was safer than eating high omega-6 vegetable oils. It is also believed that a diet high in antioxidant nutrients like beta-carotene, vitamins A, C, and E protect against all types of cancer including melanoma. Another important step towards preventing this cancer is to limit sun exposure by using sun-screen.

Oral Cancers

The incidence of cancer of the mouth, tongue and throat is quite high in India compared to western countries. It accounts for 30 to 50 per cent of all cancers in this country. This cancer can prove quite harmful because of its effect on personal appearance and the ability to eat. Men with oral cancer greatly outnumber women.

Symptoms: Oral cancers can be easily detected in an early stage. Any persistent sore on the lips, tongue, or soft tissue inside the mouth raises a suspicion of oral cancer. Other symptoms may include development of white or red patches that bleed and do not go away and painless swelling of the lymph nodes located in the neck.

Lip cancer may appear first as a growth, most often on the lower lip, that form a dry crust, which bleeds when removed and then crusts over again. Cancer of the hard palate usually manifests itself as a persistent sore, which may ulcerate. All of the oral cancers may produce mild irritation and pain, which worsen as the cancer progresses. Eventually, these pains may also be in or around the ear. Difficulty in swallowing is the most common symptom suggesting throat cancer. Initially, the problem is confined mostly to solid foods, but eventually, swallowing even pureed foods or fluids may be difficult. Often, the person describes a feeling of a chronic lump in the throat. Other symptoms are frequent spitting up of undigested food and choking. There may also be a sore throat and possible voice changes as the tumour grows.

Causes: The most important causes of oral cancer are smoking and tobacco chewing. Pipe and cigar smokers have a higher-than-normal incidence of lip cancers. Overall, tobacco users have 15 times more oral cancer than non-smokers. The risk rises to more than 50-fold among those who chew tobacco and snuff. The combination of smoking and heavy alcohol use seems to compound the risk.

Other contributing factors include nutritional deficiencies, chronic mouth infections and poor dental hygiene. Excessive sun exposure carries a risk of lip cancer.

Diagnosis: Careful physical examination inside the mouth, throat and palpating of the lymph node are necessary to check for swelling or change in consistency. Biopsy is however essential to diagnoise oral cancer.

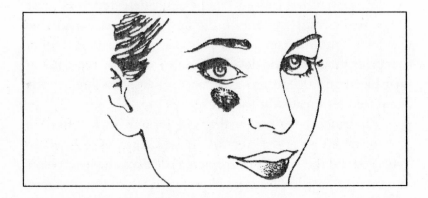

Treatment: Basically, most oral cancers are treated surgically. Another method implied is radiation therapy. It is particularly effective during the early stages of the disease. Chemotherapy can be an effective method in reducing the size and density of certain types of tumours.

Natural Methods: Natural methods can be implied to reduce pain and relieve other symptoms of cancer and after effects of medical treatment. Warm water enema may be used to detoxify the body. Other methods include daily dry friction, hip or sitz bath, relaxation techniques and meditation. Ginger-root is highly effective in preventing or minimising nausea, a common complication of radiation treatments and chemotherapy. Oral and throat cancers often interfere with normal eating. It would therefore, be necessary to take balanced diet of soft or liquid foods. Enriched liquid supplements may be necessary if the medical treatment makes it impossible to swallow.

Ovarian Cancer

Cancer of the ovary is a disease in which cancer cells are found in the ovary. Approximately 25,000 women in the United States are diagnosed with this disease each year. The ovary is a small organ in the pelvis that makes female hormones and holds egg cells which, when fertilized, can develop into a baby. There are two ovaries, one each, located on either side of the uterus.

The disease can occur at any age, but is more prevalent after menopause. There is greater risk for women who have never had children. However, women who use contraceptives are at lower risk. Unfortunately, the vast majority of women with ovarian cancer are diagnosed with advanced disease.

Symptoms: More often women with early ovarian cancer have no symptoms or very mild and non specific symptoms. However, some women get symptoms like gastrointestinal discomfort, pelvic pressure, and pain. By the time symptoms are present, women with ovarian cancer usually have advanced disease. Because cancer of the ovary may spread to the peritoneum, the sac inside the abdomen that holds the intestines, uterus, and ovaries, many women with cancer of the ovary may have fluid inside the peritoneum, which causes swelling of the abdomen. If the cancer has spread to the muscle under the lung that controls breathing, fluid may build up under the lungs and cause shortness of breath.

Causes: The specific cause of ovarian cancer is not known. It is however, believed that hereditary factors play an important role, as this type of cancer tends to run in families. Women with two or more close family members affected by ovarian cancer may be a part of a cancer family syndrome. A women with one affected close relative has a five per cent lifetime risk of ovarian cancer.

Diagnosis: Women over the age of 40 should have a thorough pelvic examination every year or two, including palpation of the ovaries. Any enlargement of an ovary raises a suspicion of cancer. Ultrasound can be used to detect the present of a mass. A definite diagnosis usually requires laparoscopy, a procedure in which a viewing tube is inserted into the pelvic cavity through a small incision near the navel, to allow examination of the ovaries and collection of biopsy samples.

Treatment: The chance of recovery and choice of treatment depend on the patient's age and general state of health, the type and size of the tumour, and the stage of the cancer.

Three kinds of treatments are available. These include surgery, radiation therapy and chemotherapy.

Natural Methods: Natural methods can be implied as a supportive therapy to intensive medical and surgical treatments. Frequent warm water enemas can be used to cleanse the bowels and remove toxins from the body. Other natural methods may include daily dry friction, neutral immersion bath, hot fomentation, deep breathing exercises, relaxation methods and meditation. These methods can help relieve symptoms of cancer and increase immune system for healing.

Nutrition plays an important role in preventing ovarian

cancer. It is believed that antioxidant vitamins A, C and E and beta carotene can help avert genetic changes in cells which promotes the development of this cancer. Foods that contain high levels of vitamins A and C and beta carotene include citrus fruits, orange and dark green vegetables and cruciferous vegetables such as broccoli, cabbage, brussels sprouts and cauliflower. Those high in vitamin E are wheat germ, vegetable oils, nuts and seeds and green vegetables. Some studies also suggest that a low fat diet may help ward off this cancer.

Pancreatic Cancer

Cancer of the pancreas is a disease in which cancer cells are found in the tissues of the pancreas. The pancreas is an oblong, pear-shaped organ, about six inches long, that lies within a loop of the small intestine behind the stomach. Pancreas produces juices that help break down food, and hormones such as insulin that regulate how the body stores and uses food.

The area of the pancreas that produces digestive juices is called the exocrine pancreas. About 95 per cent of pancreatic cancers begin in this area. The hormone-producing area of the pancreas is called the endocrine pancreas. Only about five per cent of pancreatic cancers start here.

Symptoms: The most common symptoms of pancreatic cancer are nausea, loss of appetite, unexplained loss of weight, pain in the upper or middle of the abdomen, or yellowing of the skin.

Causes: The precise cause of pancreatic cancer is not known. However, smoking has been strongly implicated as a factor because the occurrence among smokers is more than double than that of non smokers. A high meat diet too has been linked to an increased risk of pancreatic cancer. Working with dry cleaning agents, benzene and other chemicals are also believed to cause this cancer. A sudden onset of diabetes is also considered a cause for this cancer. Some studies suggest that diabetic women are at greater risk of developing this disease.

Diagnosis: Ultrasound test may be done to find tumours. A CT scan, a special type of x-ray that uses a computer to make a picture of the inside of the abdomen, may also be done. Another special scan called magnetic resonance imaging (MRI), which uses magnetic waves to make a picture of the inside of the abdomen, may be done as well. A test called an Endoscopic Retrograde Cholangio Pancreatography (ERCP) may also be done. During this test, a flexible tube is put down the throat, through the stomach, and into the small intestine. The doctor can see through the tube and inject dye into the drainage tube (duct) of the pancreas so that the area can be seen more clearly on a x-ray. During ERCP, the doctor may also put a fine needle into the pancreas to take out some cells for biopsy.

Treatment: Medically, three types of treatment are used.These are surgery, radiation therapy and chemotherapy.

Natural Method: Pain and other symptoms of cancer and the after-effects of medical treatment can be relieved through certain natural methods. These methods may include frequent warm water enemas, daily dry friction, cold hip or sitz bath, neutral immersion bath, relaxation methods and meditation. The use of biological therapy (using the body's immune system to fight cancer) is being tested in clinical trials for treating pancreatic cancer. It uses materials made by the body or made in a laboratory to boost, direct, or restore the body's natural defenses against the disease.

Prostate Cancer

Prostate cancer is one of the most common type of malignancy in men and second only to lung cancer is male cancer mortality. The prostate gland is a part of the male reproductive system. It is comparable in shape and size to a large chestnut. It measures approximately one and a half inches in width and about an inch in length and weighs approximately 25 grams. It is situated at the base of the urinary bladder and around the commencement of the urethra. The gland plays an important role in normal sexual life and its function is to secrete a fluid, which is added to semen during the sexual intercourse.

According to the Canadian Cancer Society, about 30 per cent of men develop prostate cancer, usually after age 65, and the risk becomes greater with age. It appears that certain groups are more vulnerable than others. For instance, in the United States, the incidence of prostate cancer among African-American men is 32 per cent higher than in Caucasians.

Symptoms: The first symptom of prostate cancer is difficulty in starting urination, inability to empty the bladder fully, and frequent urination, especially at night. Other symptoms are pain or burning during urination, blood in urine and dull, chronic pain in the lower back, pelvis, or upper thighs.

Causes: Abnormal reproductive and sexual patterns are generally believed to be main cause of prostate cancer. It has been established that increasingly prevalent cancer of the prostate glands in men is often caused by such unnatural practices as irregularity of or undue abstinence from sexual gratification. Unnatural practices like heavy petting which leads to a high degree of sexual excitement without the natural conclusion and the practice of withdrawal or deliberate prolongation of the sex act can contribute to prostate disorders and increase the risk of prostate cancer. A high-fat diet is also often linked to prostate cancer.

Diagnosis: It would be advisable for all men over the age of 65 to undergo annual screening for prostate cancer, starting with a digital rectal examination. For this test, a doctor inserts a gloved finger into the rectum and then feels the gland for unusual hardness or lumps. The same group also advocates that a blood test to measure prostate specific antigen (PSA, a substance secreted by prostate cells) should be done annually in addition to the digital examination, beginning at the age of 50. In case of suspicion for possible cancer, transrectal, CT scan or MRI may be necessary. However, for actual confirmation of prostate cancer, a biopsy of tissue from the suspicious areas of the gland is essential.

Treatment: The choice of treatment depends on the stage of cancer and the patient's age. Surgery, which involves removal of the prostate gland, can cure localised cancer in more than 90 per cent of cases. Surgery may be followed by radiation therapy in some cases. Hormone therapy can also be implied to treat prostate cancer. It involves a use of female hormone like estrogen to suppress male hormones, which are needed for cancer cell growth.

Natural Methods: Certain natural methods can be implied to treat pain and other symptoms of prostate cancer and to boost immune system for healing. Frequent warm water enemas are necessary to relieve toxic condition of the body. Other natural methods include daily dry friction, hot fomentation, relaxation and meditation. Hydrotherapy plays an important role as a supportive therapy. Hot and cold applications are highly beneficial in the treatment of prostate cancer. After thorough cleansing of the bowels through warm water enema, hot and cold applications may be used directly on the prostate gland and its surrounding parts. The patient should also take alternate hot and cold hip baths. The heat relieves the tissues and a brief cold immersion tones them up. These are of great value in relieving pain and reducing congestion.

Prostate cancer can be prevented by taking a low-fat vegetarian diet, as a high-fat diet has been linked to increasing risk of this type of cancer. The emphasis should be on fruits, vegetables, nuts and seeds, dried beans, peas, brown rice, and fresh juices. Foods that should be avoided are tea, coffee, alcohol, refined carbohydrates and white sugar.

The use of pumpkin seeds has been found to be an effective home remedy for prostate problems, including prostate cancer. These seeds are rich in saturated fatty acids and zinc which are essential to the health of the prostate. Other raw seeds like sunflower and sesame and raw nuts such as almonds are also great sources of unsaturated fatty acids and zinc and can therefore be used beneficially by the patient.

The use of zinc has been found valuable in several cases of prostate cancer. The patient should take about 30 mg. of this mineral daily. Vitamin E has also proved to be an important factor for prostate health. The patient should also take liberally, vitamin E-rich foods like whole grain products, green leafy vegetables, milk and all whole raw or sprouted seeds as well as Vitamin C rich foods like Indian Gooseberry (*amla*), sprouted Bengal and green grams and citrus fruits.

Skin Cancer

Skin cancer is the most prevalent malignancy. The two most common forms are basal cell carcinoma, which arises in the lowest part of the epidermis or surface layer of the skin, and squamous cell carcinoma which originates in the cells that make up the skin's outer surface. Both types are readily curable if detected early and treated properly.

Symptoms: The main symptom of skin cancer is growth or skin sores that do not heal. A basal cell cancer is typically in irregular shape. It may appear as a flat spot or a firm lump that is scaly or crusty or smooth and shiny. A squamous cell cancer also appears as scaly or crusty or smooth and shiny. It also appears as a scaly or crusty patch that may bleed occasionally. Squamous cell cancers develop most often on the rim of the ear, the mouth, and scalps of bald men.

Causes: The most common cause of skin cancer is excessive exposure to the sun's ultraviolet rays. Other risk factors are occupation exposure to coal tar, pitch, creosote, arsenic, and radium.

Diagnosis: A skin specialist often suspects skin cancer from the appearance of a sore or other lesion. However a skin biopsy is necessary for accurate diagnosis and to determine the type. These skin cancers usually do not spread to distant parts of the body, but the squamous cell type may invade nearby organs. Thus, MRI or a CT scan may be necessary if the cancer is near the eyes or other pathway to the brain.

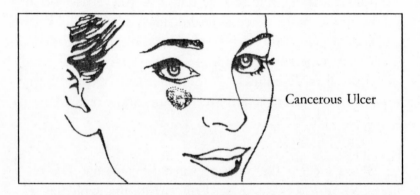

Cancerous Ulcer

Treatment: Surgery is the usual treatment for skin cancer. Radiation therapy is sometimes implied when surgical removal is not possible. Chemotherapy may also sometimes be necessary.

Natural Methods: Certain natural methods can be beneficially implied as a supportive treatment for cancer and the after effects of medical treatment. Dry friction bath will be of special value in treating this cancer as this bath opens up the pores of the body and keeps the skin in a healthy condition. Other natural methods include frequent warm water enemas, hip or sitz bath, relaxation methods and meditation. A diet that includes foods rich in antioxidants-vitamins C, E, and A or beta carotene, can help protect against cancer. Vitamin E oil applied to the affected areas may hasten healing and reduce scarring, but it should be done under medical advice.

Skin cancers can be prevented and its recurrence avoided by taking certain precautionary measures. A person should minimize exposure to the sun's ultraviolet rays as most skin cancers are caused by damage due to these rays. He should remain inside during the peak sunlight hours from 10 a.m. to 2 p.m. In case he has to go out during this period due to unavoidable reasons, he should wear a hat with a wide brim and loose-fitting but tightly woven clothing that covers most exposed skin. A sunscreen with sun protection factor should be used for remaining exposed skin.

Stomach Cancer

Cancer of the stomach, also known as gastric cancer, is a disease in which cancer cells are found in the tissues of the stomach. The stomach is a J-shaped organ in the upper abdomen where the food is digested. Food reaches the stomach through a tube called the esophagus that connects the mouth to the stomach. After leaving the stomach, partially digested food passes into the small intestine and then into the large intestine called the colon. Cancer of the stomach and bowel is more likely to occur after a person reaches forty years of age.

Symptoms: Sometimes, cancer can be in the stomach for a long time and can grow very large before it causes symptoms. In the early stages, a patient may suffer from indigestion and stomach discomfort, a bloated feeling after eating, mild nausea, loss of appetite, or heartburn. In more advanced cases, the patient may have blood in the stool, vomiting, weight loss, or pain in the stomach.

Causes: The risk of getting stomach cancer is higher if

the patient has had an infection of the stomach caused by
Helicobacter pylori, or if the patient is older, is a man, smokes
cigarettes, drinks alcoholic beverages, or frequently eats a diet
that includes lots of meat, fry and salty foods.

People who have had part of their stomach removed
sometimes develop gastric cancer 15 to 20 years later.

Diagnosis: The tests for diagnosing stomach cancer are
gastrointestinal x-ray, also known as an upper GI series or
barium meal x-ray and gastroscopy. The procedure involves
the doctor looking inside the stomach with a thin, lighted
tube called a gastroscope.

Treatment: The usual treatment for stomach cancer
involves surgical removal of the malignant tumour. This is
usually followed by chemotherapy with a combination of anti-
cancer drugs, especially if the cancer has spread beyond the
stomach.

Natural Methods: Natural methods can be implied to
relieve pain arising from medical treatments and to boost the
immune system for healing and create a feeling of well being.
These methods include repeated warm water enema, daily
dry friction bath, cold hip bath, hot fomentation, neutral
immersion bath, relaxation and meditation. The western
herbalists are also using certain herbs to minimize the side
effects of chemotherapy. These herbs include Siberian
ginseng, sarsaparilla, and wild Oregon grape, in capsule or
extract forms.

Diet restrictions are very necessary after medical
treatment. Normal eating, when possible, should be with a
liquid diet, especially fruit and vegetable juices for a few days,
before introducing solid food gradually.

Good nutrition also plays an important role in preventing
stomach cancer. A diet made up mostly of fruits, vegetables,
legumes, and whole grains can help prevent all types of
intestinal cancers. These foods are high in fibre, vitamin C

and other antioxidants, and other natural substances, which are believed to protect against cancer.

Thyroid Cancer

Cancer of the thyroid is a disease in which cancer cells are found in the tissues of the thyroid gland. The thyroid gland is situated at the base of the throat. It has two lobes, one on the right side and the other on the left. The thyroid gland makes important hormones that help the body function normally. Cancer of the thyroid is more common in women than in men. Most patients are between 25 and 65 years old.

Symptoms: Thyroid cancer typically begins as a small lump, or nodule, which can be felt while palpating the gland. Sometimes, the first obvious sign is an enlarged lymph node in the neck. As the primary thyroid tumour grows, it may spread to surrounding organs. This may result in possible voice changes, paralysis of the vocal cords and difficulty in swallowing due to a narrowing of the esophagus.

Causes: People who have been exposed to large amounts of radiation, or who have had radiation treatment for medical problems in the head and neck are at a greater risk for thyroid cancer. The cancer may not occur until 20 years or longer after radiation treatment.

Diagnosis: A doctor will feel the patient's thyroid and check for lumps in the neck. He may order blood tests and special scans to see whether a lump in the thyroid is producing too many hormones. He may also take a small amount of tissue from the thyroid for a biopsy. If cancer is confirmed, a CT scan and MRI may be done to detect any spread to nearby organs. A long X-rays may also be needed, as some thyroid cancer spreads to the lungs.

Treatment: Treatment of cancer of the thyroid depends on the type and stage of the disease, the patient's age and overall health. It is generally treated surgically. But the extent of the operation depends upon the patient's age and type of cancer. Other types of treatment are radiation therapy, chemotherapy and hormone therapy. The last-named therapy uses hormones to stop cancer cells from growing. Hormones are usually given as pills.

Natural Methods: Certain natural methods can be implied to relieve pain as well as to boost immunity. Frequent warm water enemas will help in the detoxification of the body. Other methods include daily dry friction, cold hip or sitz bath, relaxation methods and meditation.

Thyroid cancer can be prevented by avoiding exposure of the head and neck to radiation, especially during childhood. Those prone to chronic inflammation of the thyroid should undergo regular examination.

Uterine Cancer

A malignancy anywhere in the uterus or its lining is referred to as uterine cancer. The uterus is the hollow, pear-shaped organ where a baby grows. The major forms of uterine cancer are distinguished from each other by their site of origin and types of malignant cells. Cancer arising in the endometrium, the lining of the uterus, is now the most common gynecologic cancer. In the early 1900s, cervical cancer was the most prevalent form of cancer of the reproductive organs, but widespread use of the Pap smear to detect precancerous changes has greatly diminished this malignancy. Much less common are uterine sarcomas, which are cancers, made up of a type of connective tissue. Herein are discussed two major types of uterine cancer, namely endometrial and cervical cancers.

Endometrial Cancer

Cancer of the endometrium, a common kind of cancer

in women, is a disease in which cancer cells are found in the lining of the uterus, known as endometrium.

Symptoms: The main symptoms of endometrial cancer are bleeding or discharge not related to periods, difficult or painful urination, pain during sexual intercourse and pain in the pelvic area.

Causes: Typically, endometrial and other forms of uterine cancer develop following menopause. More than 75 per cent of patients are over age 50 compared to four per cent who are 40 or younger. The specific cause is not known, but estrogen is thought to be an important factor, as it stimulates growth of the endometrium. Before menopause, the levels of estrogen, progesterone, and other hormones fluctuate during the menstrual cycle, resulting in shedding of the endometrium during menstruation. But if it is exposed only to estrogen, the endometrium grows unchecked. The resulting hyperplasia is believed to set the stage for cancer.

Diagnosis: To diagnoise this cancer, the doctor will feel for any lumps or changes in the shape of the uterus and carry out same test as for cervical cancer. If the pap test does

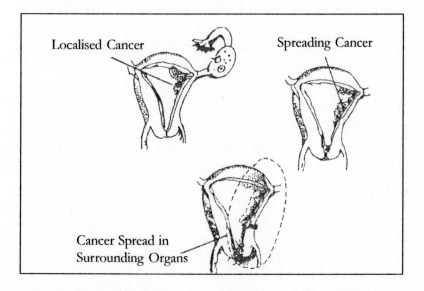

Localised Cancer   Spreading Cancer

Cancer Spread in
Surrounding Organs

not show results, a doctor may also do a dilation and curettage (D and C) or a similar test, to remove pieces of the lining of the uterus.

Treatment: The chance of recovery and choice of treatment depend on the stage of the cancer, as to whether the cancer is just in the endometrium or has spread to other parts of the uterus or other parts of the body and the general health of the patient. Medical treatments for endometrium cancer consist of surgery, radiation therapy, chemotherapy, and hormone therapy, using female hormones to kill cancer cells. Surgery, however, is the most common treatment for this cancer.

Natural Methods: Certain natural methods can be implied to relieve pain, other symptoms of cancer and the after effects of medical treatment. These methods include dry friction, hip bath, hot fomentation, relaxation methods and meditation.

Diet plays an important role in the prevention of endometrial cancer, according to researchers at the University of Alabama School of Public Health in Birmingham. A comparison of the diets of women who did and did not have endometrial cancer showed that those who ate carrots, spinach, broccoli, melon or lettuce, which are high in carotene, at least once a day were only 27 per cent as likely to have the cancer as women who ate those foods less than once a week. Eating yogurt, cheese and other calcium-rich foods also reduced the risk significantly. Meditation and relaxation technique can control the intense pain associated with advanced cancer.

Cervical Cancer

Cancer of the cervix, a common kind of cancer in women between the age of 40 and 55, is a disease in which cancer cells are found in the tissues of the cervix. The cervix is the opening of the uterus or womb. The cervix connects the uterus to the vagina.

Symptoms: Cancer of the cervix usually grows slowly over a period of time. Before cancer cells are found on the cervix, the tissues of the cervix go through changes in which cells that are not normal begin to appear. A Pap smear will usually find these cells. Later, cancer cells start to grow and spread more deeply into the cervix and to surrounding areas.

Causes: The precise cause of cervical cancer is not known. According to some studies, certain factors like beginning sexual intercourse before the age of 18, having multiple sex partners, contracting genital warts and tobacco use can contribute to this type of cancer. Other studies suggest that the use of oral contraceptives and a lack of folic acid can lead to this cancer.

Studies conducted in the 1960s and 1970s found that post-menopausal woman who took estrogen replacement alone had a greatly increased incidence of endometrial cancer, as did woman who had entered menopause late, those who had never had a baby, and those with polycystic ovaries and hormonal disorders resulting in high estrogen production.

Obesity is another major risk factor Woman who are 50 or more pounds overweight have a ninefold increase in uterine cancer, compared to woman of normal weight. Here too, estrogen is important, as it can be produced in fat tissues, even after menopause. Genetics also may play a role, because uterine cancer tends to run in families.

Diagnosis: Since there are usually no symptoms associated with cancer of the cervix, a series of tests are required to find it out. The first of these is a Pap smear, which is done by using a piece of cotton, a brush, or a small wooden stick to gently scrape the outside of the cervix in order to pick up cells. Pressure is sometimes felt, but is usually not

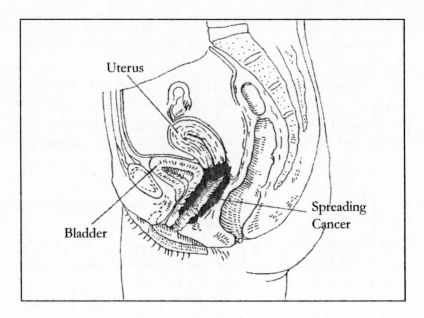

accompanied by pain. If abnormal cells are found, a sample of tissue is cut for biopsy.

Treatment: The chance of recovery and choice of treatment depend on the stage of the cancer (whether it is just in the cervix or has spread to other places) and the patient's general health.

Medically, three kinds of treatment are used. These are surgery, radiation therapy, and chemotherapy.

Natural Methods: Natural methods can be employed to control pain and other symptoms of cervical cancer as well as the after effects of medical treatments. These methods include frequent warm water enemas to cleanse the bowels and detoxify the body. Other methods may include daily dry friction, friction sitz bath, meditation and relaxation techniques, especially shavasana.

The patient should take a well-balanced diet, with emphasis on alkaline foods especially fresh fruits, raw and lightly cooked vegetables and sprouted seeds. The emphasis should also be on greens and dried beans which are high in folic acid. This can stop the virus which can lead to cervical cancer. About 80 per cent of all cases of cervical cancer occur in women infected with the virus. However, women who have high levels of folic acid in their red blood cells are much less likely to develop this cancer, according to new research by Charles Butterworth, Jr., M.D., of the University of Alabama at Birmingham. His study of 464 women infected with the virus found that those with lower levels of folic acid were five times more likely to develop cell changes leading to cervical cancer, than those with higher folic acid levels.

Eating tomatoes also appears to prevent precancerous signs of cervical cancer; namely an inflammation called Cervical Intraepithelial Neoplasia (CIN). Researchers at the University of Illinois at Chicago found that women with the highest blood levels of lycopene, of which tomatoes are the primary source, had a five times lower risk of developing the precancerous condition as compared to those who had the lowest blood levels of lycopene. Lycopene is also found in abundance in watermelon.

SOME SPECIFIC CLAIMS ABOUT CANCER CURES

11

Diet now occupies the most prominent place in the treatment of cancer. Emphasis is being placed upon mineral-vitamin rich foods, in combination with bland and non-irritating foods. These are particularly true in case of gastric and intestinal cancer. Herein are mentioned some claims made by patients, who suffered from one type of cancer or the other, about their success in curing themselves through the use of certain specific foods.

Carrot Juice

Mary C. Hogle, a graduate of the University of Kansas and an experienced student of nutrition and food chemistry, claims to have been cured by a carrot juice regime, in combination with bland foods, when it had been thought she was incurable. In her book, *Food that Alkalize and Heal,* she gives a short history of her case and some very fine suggestions on what to eat and how to prepare certain broths and bland foods. She heartily endorses carrot juice as one of the most potent alkalizers. She says, "The excellence of carrot juice as a source of vitamin A, no doubt explains much of its health value. Vitamin A has been called the anti-infective vitamin and it has as its specific function the resisting and correcting of all infection of the epithelial surfaces, which include the skin covering, the mucous membranes and all the glands. Vitamin A is considered one of the main elements, in a basic way, to protect all infections."

She further says about carrot "Carrot juice has established itself as the peer of all as a rapid alkalizer. This is no doubt partly because the contained alkalies are easily appropriated by the body and partly because juice can generally be consumed in large quantities without unpleasant or harmful effects."

Mrs. Hogle states, that the rapidity with which carrot juice corrects acid conditions has been many times demonstrated, and that acid stomach responds quickly to carrot juice. The condition of acid mouth, which produces "pink tooth brushes," can also be speedily corrected by taking carrot juice. She also states that inflammation of the eyes is speedily cleared up with the use of copious amounts of carrot juice, and that urine, many times more acidic than normal, can be returned to normal within a few hours, by drinking carrot juice copiously.

Grape Cure

About 125 years ago, Dr. Lambe, a pioneer reformer and dietitian, treated cancer in England with grapes. In recent times, Johanna Brandt, discovered for herself that cancer could be treated successfully with exclusive grape diet. She made this discovery while experimenting on her self by fasting and dieting alternately in the course of her nine-year battle against cancer. She claimed to have cured herself by this mode of treatment. The effectiveness of exclusive grape diet in treating cancer is attributable to the presence of generous quantities of salts of potash in grapes. It has been noted that there is a marked deficiency of potash in the average cancer patient.

An exclusive grape diet is thus valuable in cancer. Johanna Brandt, the author of 'Grape Cure', has given directions for this mode of treatment in her book. She recommends fasting on pure water for two or three days so as to prepare the system for the change of diet. During this period, the patient should drink plenty of pure cold water and take lukewarm water enema daily, with the strained juice of lemon.

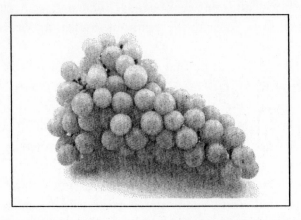

After the short fast, the patient should have a grape meal every two hours from 8 a.m. to 8 p.m. This should be followed for a week or two, even a month or two, in chronic cases of long standing. The patient should begin the grape cure with a small quantity. In course of time, about 200 grams may safely be taken at a meal. Johanna Brandt recommends the consumption of not more than two kgs of grapes daily, under most circumstances. Many varieties of grapes may be used to break the monotony of the diet. The patient may lose strength under the grape diet and the complete fast, but it is due to the presence of poisons in the system. The patient regains his strength and even puts on weight in some cases, with the same diet, after the poisons are expelled. After the exclusive grape diet the return to normal diet should be gradual.

Raw Foods

Dr. Kirstine Nolfi, M.D. of Denmark, who herself suffered from cancer of the breast, found by experiment, the value of raw foods in treating cancer. She recovered from this dreaded disease after treating herself with an exclusive raw food diet and then opened an institution called Humlegarden. She attained great success in treating cancer patients at this institution and wrote a book about her success.

In the winter of 1940-41, Dr. Nolfi was diagnosed as having cancer but she refused treatment by X-ray, radium and surgery. Because of her refusal to accept established, approved medical treatment, she was persecuted until she ceased her medical practice. However, she successfully treated herself with an exclusive raw food diet and regained her health. After recovery, she opened an establishment at Humlegarden. Here, she treated many cancer and other patients.

In her book, Dr. Nolfi tells how, whenever she slipped off her raw food diet or used salt, the condition reappeared. Then, when she resumed and stuck to the raw food diet, the cancer subsided. This experience shows that cancer cannot be cured but it can be prevented and held under control by a raw juice and raw food diet. Dr. Nolfi gave a great deal of credit to raw garlic and raw potatoes, which she claims were the key vegetables in the success of the raw food diet.

About 1000 patients visited the sanitorium annually and not only the patients were on a raw food diet but all members of the hospital staff lived entirely on foods which were not heat treated.

Wheat Grass

Wheat grass is a wonder plant. Dr. Ann Wigmore of Boston, U.S., the founder director of the Hippocrates Health Institute, and well-known naturopath and pioneer in the field of living food nutrition, tested the effect of a drink made of fresh wheat grass in the treatment of leukaemia. She claims to have cured several cases of this disease by this method.

According to Dr. Ann Wigmore, "guided by spiritual mentality and nourished only by live uncooked food, the body will run indefinitely, unhampered by sickness." Dr. G.H. Earp Thomas, a scientist and soil expert, isolated over one hundred elements from fresh wheat grass and concluded that it is a complete food.

The juice extracted from fresh wheat grass is considered beneficial in the treatment of cancer. By furnishing the body with live minerals, vitamins, trace elements and chlorophyll, the wheatgrass juice may help to repair the damaged cells.

An exclusive diet of wheat grass can be used beneficially in treating diseases. In adopting this mode of treatment, the patient should undertake fasting on wheat grass, for seven days. This fast provides the body with all the nutrients of the richest living food in a form so concentrated and easy to digest that it provides virtually all the benefits of a complete fast with none of the dangers of total abstinence. Such a fast can cleanse and nourish at the same time. One can be confident of complete safety and real health-building results.

To prepare for the wheat grass fast, it is essential for the patient to undertake repeated warm water enema so as to cleanse the body of accumulated waste products. It is necessary to eliminate this putrefaction. The wheat grass fast consists of three or four wheat grass juice drinks each days plus two chlorophyll implants. If the patient does not like the taste or odour of the juice, he can take four implants instead of two, with same beneficial results.

Upon awakening, the patient should drink two glasses of warm water, mixed with the juice of one lemon sweetened with molasses or honey. Then, the colon should be thoroughly cleansed with an enema to eliminate any debris clinging to the inner walls of the colon. The patient should sip 120 ml of pure wheat grass chlorophyll three times a day, at five-hourly intervals. Each drink may be diluted with water on 50:50 basis. While on wheat grass therapy, the patient should drink at least one litre of not-too-cold water each day, placing a small bunch of wheat grass in each drink to purify it.

The role of nutrition in cancer has been confirmed by new scientific observations which recognise the fact that the blood lacks in organic mineral elements and true nutrients out of which true, healthy, vibrant cells are created. The blood and consequently, the tissues, have become so saturated with waste and foreign matter that the life of the individual is being threatened. As a safety measure, the body builds the cancerous cells from the blood pollutants at a rapid pace, reducing the impurities in the blood. During the wheat grass therapy, the growths are brought, piecemeal, into the bloodstream and removed through the eliminative organs. The therapy consists of grass chlorophyll cocktails and live food taken in an atmosphere of happiness and thankfulness.

PREVENTION OF CANCER

12

A great shift in Cancer Research occurred in the 1990s. During the previous two decades, the modern medical system had failed to find a cure in the fight against cancer. In the mean time, the rate of deaths from cancer continued to rise. Research studies for cancer thus, shifted towards prevention rather than cure of the disease. It aims at eliminating the causative agents.

This shift clearly vindicates the opinions expressed by ancient physicians on cancer. The eminent Persian physician, Avicenna stated long back that advanced cases of cancer would not cure. This physician, as well as other eminent physicians of the past, laid emphasis on the dietary treatment of the disease. Major cancer research studies have now concentrated on the course suggested by these physicians.

It is thus, more important to prevent the disease than treat it. The measures to treat the disease bring only temporary results and a poor survival rate.

Imparting Education

The most important aspect of prevention of cancer is to impart proper education to people about factors that cause cancer. Thus, for instance, the incidence of mouth cancer is the highest in India and forms one-third of all the cancer cases in this country. This is mainly due to widely-prevalent habit of chewing tobacco. Those who are in the habit of chewing tobacco daily, run eight times more risk of developing mouth cancer than do the non-chewers. The risk is even higher when chewing tobaccos started at an earlier age. Substantial reducation in the incidence of mouth cancers can be achieved by giving up the tobacco-chewing habit completely.

Giving up Smoking

The incidence of cancer of the lung has also been steadily increasing in India. The most important cause of this cancer is cigarette smoking. Sutdies have shown that there is a clear relationship between the number of cigarettes smoked and the incidence of lung cancer. The longer a cigarette is, the more tar and nicotine one inhales. The last half of the cigarette contains twice as much tar and nicotine as the first half. The susceptibility to this type of cancer, can be reduced proprtionate to the number of years that smoking has been given up.

Avoiding Early Marriages and Multiple Pregnancies

Cancer of the uterine cervix, which is quite frequent among women in this country, can also be controlled substantially. This cancer is mainly caused by early marriage and multiple pregnancies. By avoiding these, this cancer can be prevented to a great extent. Other helpful measures for preventing cancer are improvement of personal hygiene such as of mouth, skin and genitals; control of air pollution; testing of all drugs, cosmetics, and food additives for possible cancer causing substances; special efforts to reduce radiation to the minimum without reducing the benefits derived therefrom; enforcement of measures to protect workers from carcinogenic agents in industries and avoidance of use of various types of pesticides. The incidence of cancer can thus, be prevented to a considerable extent by avoiding smoking cigarettes, excessive drinking of alcohol, excessive exposure to sun, indiscriminate use of birth control pills and early and unnatural sexual intercourse. The most important factor to prevent all types of cancers is drastic changes in diet. The measures in this connection, should include avoiding all flesh foods, eating liberally green vegetables, fresh fruits, cereal brans, dried beans, regular intake of raw vegetable salad, liberal intake of nuts especially almonds and taking a low calorie diet.

Building up Body's Defense System through Excellent Nutrition

The best way to prevent cancer is to build up the body's defenses through excellent nutrition. This can be achieved by completely avoiding all refined, synthetic and processed foods, white, flour, enriched fortified foods, white sugar, all frozen, bottled and tinned foods and foods with chemical additives. The foods, which build up the body and strengthen the immune system, are natural, whole foods, raw vegetables and fruits, protein from vegetable sources, milk, whole grains and vitamins and minerals in their natural form.

A survey of the dietary habits of Chinese people between 1973-1984, was conducted by researchers to ascertain what diseases they developed. They found, among other things, that people who ate more sulphur-rich vegetables, including cabbage, broccoli, cauliflower, garlic and onions had the lowest risks of cancer, in general.

Liberal Intake of Foods Rich in Antioxidants

Antioxidants may also help reduce the incidence of cancer. They act as protective substances by destroying free radicals, which are the harmful by-products formed through the body's metabolism. Free radicals damage cells and initiate carcinogenesis which is the development of cancerous cells.

Vitamin C, beta carotene (precursor of vitamin A), vitamin E and selenium are all antioxidants. In addition, there are hundreds more naturally occurring antioxidants found in plant foods.

Studies have shown that antioxidants work best when combined and that the presence of fibre and other plant compounds may provide additional health benefits. It is therefore advisable to get antioxidants from our diet rather than relying on supplements. Foods rich in vitamin C are citrus fruits, green leafy vegetables, Indian goosebery and sprouted Bengal and green grams. vitamin A is found in whole milk, curds, butter, green leafy vegetables, yellow fruits and vegetables. Valuable sources of vitamin E are wheat or cereal germ, whole grain products, vegetable oils, green leafy vegetables, milk and whole and sprouted seeds. Selenium is found in Brewer's yeast, garlic, onions, tomatoes and milk.

Dietary guidelines

For prevention of cancer, The American Cancer Society has developed the folowing dietary guideines:

1. Choose most of the foods you eat from plant sources. Eat at least five servings of fruits and vegetables each day.

2. Include other plant foods such as breads, cereals, grain products, rice and dried beans wih every meal. These foods are all excellent sources of vitamins, minerals and fibre.

3. Limit your intake of high fat foods. Low fat vegetarian foods include skim milk products, cooked dry peas and beans, whole grain breads and cereals, fruits and vegetables. Added fats like butter, margarine, oil and mayonnaise should be avoided since it only increases the total fat in the diet. Whenever possible select low-fat or non-fat food produts. Also, choose most of

the foods you eat from plant sources since these foods have little or no fat. You should attempt to reduce fat intake to 20-30 per cent of total calories.

4. Limit consumption of alcoholic beverages.

Avoiding Contact with Carcinogens

There are certain types of cancers which are associated with definite occupations, habits, customs and usage. These cancers can be prevented by avoiding contact with carcinogens which cause them and by taking precautions at work sites. Periodic examination and clinical test after certain age will go a long way in early detection, prevention and treatment of cancers.

Natural and Simple Lifestyle

The other preventive measures are regular physical exercise and yogic asanas, plenty of fresh and pure air, plenty of rest, adequate sleep, relaxation and meditation and complete freedom from worries and mental stress.

13

TREATMENT CHART FOR CANCER

Diet

1. Raw juice diet for five days. Take a glass of fresh fruit or vegetable juice, diluted with water in a 50:50 ratio, every two hours from 8 a.m. to 8 p.m. Fruits and vegetables which may be used for juicing are apple, pineapple, papaya, grapes, orange, carrot, spinach and beet. Citrus fruit juices or green vegetable juices will be especially beneficial. During the period of juice fast, warm water enema should be used daily to cleanse the bowels and detoxify the body. In advanced cases of cancer, repeated warm water enemas will be beneficial.

2. An exclusive diet of fresh fruits for further five days. In this regimen, take three meals a day of fresh juicy fruits mentioned above at five-hourly intervals.

3. Thereafter, gradually adopt a well-balanced diet on the following lines:

   1. *Upon arising:* A glass of lukewarm water with half a freshly-squeezed lime and a teaspoon of honey.

   2. *Breakfast:* Fresh fruits such as apple, grapes, pear, peach, pineapple, papaya and a glass of milk, preferably raw-goat's milk, sweetened with honey and some seeds or nuts, especially almonds or sesame seeds.

   3. *Lunch:* A bowl of freshly prepared steamed vegetables such as carrot, cabbage, cauliflower,

bottle gourd, ridge gourd and beans, two or three whole wheat chapatis or brown rice and a glass of butter milk.

4. *Mid-afternoon:* A glass of beet juice mixed with green vegetable juice on 50:50 basis.

5. *Dinner:* A large bowl of salad of fresh raw vegetables such as lettuce, carrot, cabbage, cucumber, tomato, radish, red beet, onion and sprouts such as alfalfa and mung beans with lime juice and olive oil dressing. This may be followed by a vegetable soup and whole meal bread, if desired.

6. *Bedtime snack:* A glass of milk or one fruit.

Note: The short juice fast followed by an all-fruit diet may be repeated at monthly intervals.

Avoid: Tea, coffee, sugar, white flour, all products made with sugar and white flour, all refined foods, fried foods and flesh foods as well as condiments, pickles, alcohol and smoking. Salt should be taken in very minute quantity. All environmental sources of carcinogens, such as smoking and carcinogenic chemicals in air, water and food should be eliminated.

Especially Beneficial

Beet juice, cabbage, carrot, citrus fruits, curd, garlic, olive oil, milk, brown rice, soyabeans, tomato, watermelon and wheat bran.

Other Measures

1. Fresh air, breathing and other light exercises.
2. Adequate rest, proper sleep relaxation and meditation.
3. Avoid mental worries and stress.

GLOSSARY

Androgen	:	A male hormone
Aromatic amine	:	A chemical substance derived from petroleum products, which may cause cancer
Benign	:	A tumour or tissue which is not cancerous and does not spread
Bone marrow	:	A spongy tissue in the middle of bones that makes blood cells
Carcinogen	:	A substance which produces malignant growth or cancer
Carcinoma	:	A malignant tumour arising in an epithelial tissue
Cell	:	The basic unit of which the body is made
Chemotherapy	:	Treatment of cancer by drugs
Colicky pain	:	A severe pain which increases in spasms
Colon	:	A part of the large intestine
CT scan	:	A computerised X-ray, which gives a very clear picture
Dilation	:	Excessive enlargement of an organ
Duodenum	:	The part of the intestine
Endocrine glands	:	Glands that secrete hormones into the bloodstream
Endometrium	:	Lining of uterus

Enzymes	:	Secretion of the special cells of the body for digestion of foods
Epidermis	:	A surface layer of the skin
Epithelium	:	The lining that covers the internal and external surfaces of the body
ERCP (Endoscopic retrograde cholangio pancreatography)	:	A method to have a clear view of the pancreatic area by injecting dye through the tube put into the small intestine
Esophagus	:	The gullet; a tube connecting the pharynx or throat with the stomach
Estrogen	:	Hormone secreted by ovaries
Gastroscopy	:	Use of a flexible lighted instrument, which is swallowed to examine the inside of the stomach and upper part of the small bowel
Genetic	:	Inherited
Hepatitis	:	A virus transmitted through the blood, causing inflammation of the liver
Hodgkin's	:	A type of lymphoma named after the doctor who first diagnoised it
Hormone	:	A chemical substance secreted in the blood from the endocrine glands
Laparotomy	:	An exploratory abdominal operation
Laproscopy	:	Examination of ovaries and collection of biopsy samples through a viewing tube inserted into the pelvic cavity
Leukaemia	:	Malignant conditions in which abnormal cells are present in the blood and bone marrow

Lymph Node	:	Nodules of tissue in the lymph channels that make lymphocytes and filter out unwanted substances
Lymphatic system	:	Circulatory network of lymph-carrying vessels and the lymph nodes
Malignant	:	A tumour or tissue which is cancerous and spreads
Metastasis	:	Spread of cancer from one part of the body to another
Menopause	:	Cessation of menstruation
MRI	:	A specetial test which uses a magnet to make a picture of the inside of the organ:
Mutation	:	A permanent change in generic material DNA
Neoplasm	:	A tumour or new growth, malignant or benign
Nodule	:	A small swelling or aggregation of cells
Oncogen	:	A substance that produces cancer
Oncology	:	The term for study of tumour
Organ	:	Aggregation or collection of tissues
Palpate	:	To feel by hand
Smear	:	Scrapping of cells from the cervix of the uterus for biopsy
Portal system	:	Vessels that carry the blood that drains from the intestine to the liver
Platelets	:	Kind of cells in the blood that help it to clot
Polyp	:	A benign outgrowth of tissue
Primary cancer	:	A cancer present at the site in

which it originated

Progesterone	:	A naturally occurring hormone secreted by the ovary
Prognosis	:	A prediction about the course of a disease and chances of recovery
PSA (Prostate specific antigen)	: :	A substance secreted by prostate cells
Radioactive	:	Substances that emit X-rays
Radiation therapy	:	Use of high-dose X-rays or other high energy rays to kill cancer cells and shrink tumour
Sarcoma	:	Malignant tumour arising in connective tissue likes bone, cartilage and muscle
Surgery	:	Medical treatment in which a surgeon cuts open your body to remove the cancer.
Terminal cancer	:	Cancers that may, more or less prove fatal
Tissue	:	A collection or mass of cells of one kind
Ultrasound	:	Sound waves of a frequency which are beyond hearing

Indian Names of Foods Stuffs & Herbs mentioned in the Book

English	Hindi	Bengali	Gujarati	Kannada	Malayalam	Marathi	Tamil	Telugu
Almond	Badam	Badam	Badam	Badam	Badam	Badam	Badam	Badam
Apple	Seb	Seu	Safarjan	Seleu	Apple	Safarchand	—	Amruta
Beet root	Chukandar	Beet	Beet	Beet	Beet	Beet	Beet	Beet
Brussel sprouts	Chotee gobee	Bilati-band hakopi	—	Mara kosu	—	—	Kalakose	—
Cabbage	Bandgobhi	Bandha kopi	Kobi	Kosu	Mutta gosa	Kobi	Muttaikose	Gos koora
Carrot	Gajor	Gajor	Gajor	Gajjare	Carrot	Gajar	Carrot	Gajjara
Cauliflower	Phul gobi	Phul gobi	Phul gobi	Hokosu	—	Phul gobi	Kovippu	—
Celery	Ajivain-ka-patta	Pandhumi sag	Ajmana pan	—	Sellary	—	—	—
Colchicum	Hirantutuya	—	—	—	—	—	—	—
Cucumber	Khira	Sasha	Kakdi	Southe kayi	Vellarikka	Kakadi	Kakkarikkai	Dosa kaye
Curd	Dahi	Doyi	Dahi	Mosaru	Thayire	Dahi	Thayir	Perygu
Fenugreek	Methi	Methi	Methi	Menthe	Uluva	Methi	Venthiya Kerrai	Menthikee
Garlic	Lahasoon	Rashun	Lasan	Bellulli	Vellulli	Lasson	Vllipoondu	Vellulli
Ginger	Adrak	Ada	Adu	Shunti	Inji	Ale	Iriji	Allam
Grapes	Angoor	Angoor	Draksha	Draksha	Mundiringa	Draksha	Draksha	Draksha

Indian Names of Foods Stuffs & Herbs mentioned in the Book

English	Hindi	Bengali	Gujarati	Kannada	Malayalam	Marathi	Tamil	Telugu
Grape-fruit	Chakotra	Bilati batabi	Chakotra	—	Mundri pazham	Bedaana	—	—
Green-grams	—	Mug	Mug	Kesare kalu	Cheru payaree	Mung	Pcesipayir	Pasalu
Guava	Amrud	Payra	Jamphal	Seeba	Perakka	Peru	Koya pazham	Jami pa
Holy basil	—	Tulsi	Tulsi	Vishpu tulsi	Trittaua	Tulshi	Thulasi	Thulasi
Indian gooseberry	Amla	Amlaki	Amla	Nellikai	Nellikai	Anvla	Nellikai	Vsirikayi
Lettuce	Salad patta	Salad pata	Salat	Hakkarike-soppu	Uvarcheera	—	—	—
Lime	Nimboo	Lebu	Kadgi	Nimbe	Cherunag-anga	Musumbe	Elumichai	Nimmpapa
Linseed	Alsi	Tishi	Alsi	—	Cheruchana vithu	Jawas	Ali vidai	Auise ginzalu
Liquorice	—	Jasthi madu	Jethi	Sashti-madhu	Iratimadhur	Jyeshnash	Attimadhu-ram	Lashti
Margosa	—	Nim	Limbro	Beslu	Vepa	Nimba	Veppa	Vepa
Mint	—	Pudina	Pudina	Pudina	Pudina	Pudina	Pudina	Pudina

Indian Names of Foods Stuffs & Herbs mentioned in the Book

English	Hindi	Bengali	Gujarati	Kannada	Malayalam	Marathi	Tamil	Telugu
Orange	Narangi/	Kamala lebu sangtra	Santra	Kithilai	Madhurana-ranga	santre	Kichili pazham	Kamala pandu
Papaya	Papita	Pepe	Papaya	Pharangi	Omakai	Popai	Pappali	Boppayi pandu
Parsley	Prajmoda	—	—	Achu morha	Kuthambe-lari	—	—	—
Peach	Arhu	Peach	Peech	Marasebu	Pochad poxam	Peech	Aru	—
Pear	Naspati	Nashapti	Nashati	Berikai	Sabarjil	Nashpati	Berikai	Berikai
Pineapple	Ananas	Anarash	Ananas	Ananas	Kayitha chakka	Ananas	Anasi pazham	Anasa Paue
Soya-bean	Bhat	Garikalia	—	—	—	—	—	—
Spinach	Palak	Palang sag	Palak	Basala-soppu	Basala cheera	Palak	Pasalaikeeri	Bachahali koora
Tomato	Tamator	Tamater	Tameton	Tomatoha-nnu	Thakkali	Belwangi	Semitekkali	Seema vankaya
Turmeric	Haldi	Holud	Haldhar	Anashina	Manjal	Halad	Manjal	Pasupu
Watermelon	Tarbuz	Tarmuj	Tarbuj	Kallangadi	Thannir mathan	Kalingad	Darbusini	Puchakayi

BIBLIOGRAPHY

Jean Carper, Food Your Miracle Medicine, London: Simon and Schuster, First edition, 1995.

Health Research, Is Cancer Curable Washington, 1969

Max Gerson, A Cancer Therapy, New York: Gerson Institute in association with Station Hill press, Fifth edition, 1990.

Paavo Airola, Cancer the total approach, Oregon: Health Plus Publishers, fifteenth edition 1993.

Bakhru H.K., Natural Home Remedies for Common Ailments, New Delhi: Orient Paperback, Sixth Printing, 1999.

V.N. Bhave, N.S. Deodhar, S.V. Bhava, You and Your Health, New Delhi: National Book Trust, Second Edition 1983.

Paul Bergner, Healing Power of Garlic, New Delhi, Orient Paperback 1998.

Reader's Digest, Guide to Medical Cures and Treatments, Montreal, The Reader's Digest Association (Canada) Ltd.